Luna Yoga

Vital Fertility and Sexuality

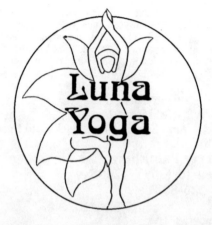

Luna Yoga

Vital Fertility and Sexuality

Adelheid Ohlig

Translated from the German by Meret Liebenstein

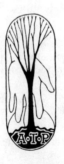

Ash Tree Publishing
Woodstock, New York

Original title *LunaYoga* © Adelheid Ohlig
English translation by Meret Liebenstein
Edited and adapted by Amy Sophia Marashinsky and Susun Weed

©1994 by **Ash Tree Publishing**
PO Box 64, Woodstock, NY 12498
phone/FAX 914-246-8081

Typesetting by Kimberley Eve
Illustrations by Esther Lisette Ganz ,
    except pages 65, 165 by Kimberley Eve
Cover art by Kimberley Eve

Library of Congress Catalog Card Number 94-71324
ISBN 096146206X

Publisher's Cataloging in Publication

Ohlig, Adelheid
    [LunaYoga. English]
    Luna yoga : Vital Fertility and Sexuality / by
Adelheid Ohlig ; translated by Meret Liebenstein ; notes by Susun Weed.
    p. cm. -- (Best of Europe)
    Translation of: LunaYoga.
    Includes bibliographical references.
    ISBN 0-9614620-6-X

1. Yoga, Hatha. 2. Women--Health and hygiene. 3. Fertility, Human.
I. Title. II. Series
RA781.7.03513 1994   613.7'046'082   QBI94-1144

For love and lust and for desire
For passion and for playfulness
With the courage of the lion
The power of the lioness

Table of Contents

PART FOUR
LUNA YOGA Healing Sequences/121

PART FIVE
Sensuous and Sensible Additions/135

PART SIX
The End, and the Beginning/181

Introduction

My Yoga practice, once so intense, has fallen off in past years, as I have been involved in parenting an extraordinary child as well as maintaining a multifaceted career. When my hormones began "acting up" a couple of years ago, my face started itching and wouldn't stop no matter what treatment I applied (acupuncture, herbs, relaxation, bodywork, creams). One day at the end of my rope with frustration and dis-ease, I pleaded with the universe for help, and the voice inside whispered in no uncertain terms: "Stand on your head for five minutes a day." Within a week of following these inner instructions, the condition that had afflicted me for two months was completely gone, without a single recurring symptom. Is it any wonder that this powerful medicine called Yoga is also a way of life?

Even before I heard her personal story which is so like my own, I was already stunned by the title of Adelheid Ohlig's work: *Luna Yoga*. She began studying to be a Yoga teacher in Germany in 1978; in 1978 I also began to teach what I called "Luna Yoga" in Berkeley, California. Following my intuition, I focused not on form, but on the subtle movements of healing energy through the body and the development of awareness of this moving force. I especially enjoyed working with women's sexuality and the "female blood mysteries" which I came to understand as being at the center of the shamanic and yogic work I would teach for the next twenty years. An underlying premise of my book, *Shakti Woman*, is that if women could only reclaim our sacred menstruation rites, we would regain our ancient empowerment.

My work is anchored in knowledge of the ancient matristic cultures documented by Marija Gimbutas in *The Civilization of the Goddess*. I have taken heart from the fact that female sexuality and the healing arts appear to have been at the center of their social organization. From the artifacts it is clear that women invented Yoga millennia before it was codified and written down in India in its present form. It is this knowledge that lives in our bodies even today and can be awakened through yogic practices and feminist empowerment. My gradual authority in this work came through my own powerful self-healing process, a miracle of transformation that made my sick body well and brought about an integration that made my life worth living.

Likewise, Ohlig's work is all about awakening healing energies and feminist body awareness. Ohlig also came to her work through a healing crisis—in her case, an even more serious one, cervical cancer. Her intuitive choice to forgo western treatments (such as surgery, radiation or chemo-therapy) led to an awakening of her inner certainty and trust that would sustain her in a disciplined two-year course of focused yogic study. Her commitment to the body's natural process of healing itself has given her a deep sense of knowing and personal authority that vibrates through her written work, even in translation. Her courage inspires, and her unleashed creativity is a vivid demonstration of the freedom of movement she claims is necessary for women's health.

Like myself, Ohlig places the roots of Yoga in the ancient Goddess traditions of the Paleolithic and Neolithic times. The key is the women's blood mysteries, with their natural integration of sexuality, creative expression, and healing power. She feels strongly that the imposition of patriarchal menstrual taboos and sexual inhibitions have led inevitably to the diseases afflicting modern women, and it is toward letting go of these unnatural restrictions that her release work is aimed.

Through combining simple Yoga and breathing exercises, self-love, tribal fertility dance movements, and a sound application of the principles developed by Aviva Steiner for female reproductive health, Ohlig's *Luna Yoga* is an integrated path for women to achieve a healthy, balanced life.

Reading this book was more than enjoyable; it touched me at my center. I remembered my own deep Yoga, and I was reminded and reassured of the living foundation of sisterhood that exists among women as we open to and share the knowledge that lives within our bodies. Yoga isn't just a set of physical exercises, or a way to stay young or thin, or a "stress reduction" program. It's a profound, mystical, non-rational method of healing—that is to say, curing—the body of illness and disease. And Ohlig's approach to Yoga (unlike most) is integrated with basic feminist principles as well as tribal methods of right-living in the body. It's a tiny little manifesto for the modern woman, with step-by-step instructions for how to reclaim herself.

Vicki Noble, feminist healer, co-creator of
Motherpeace Tarot, and author of
Shakti Woman: Feeling Our Fire, Healing Our World

Publisher's Preface

LUNA YOGA seized me as soon as I encountered it. I was in Germany teaching at a conference. So was Adelheid. A student of Yoga for more than twenty-five years, I went to Adelheid's class expecting the ususal breathing, stretching, meditating. What a delightful surprise to find myself in the midst of a quiet revolution in the way Yoga is offered to women.

It took me less than twenty-four hours to discover that Adelheid had written a book and to propose to her that Ash Tree Publishing bring this vital work to American women as part of our Best of Europe series. She agreed, with pleasure.

Five years have passed since then. Working out rights and royalties, finding a translator, retranslating the translation, adapting the presentation to American women, designing, typesetting (and typesetting and typesetting), and communicating across the ocean and across languages—these tasks have sometimes seemed endless, especially this past year, when Amy and Kimberley and I have lived, breathed, and done virtually nothing but craft LUNA YOGA.

Today we are done. With tremors of delicious excitement I now release LUNA YOGA from my hands and place it in yours. May this knowledge help you, as it has helped so many others, to greater self-love and wellbeing.

It is begun in beauty; it is done in beauty; it is ended in beauty.

Susun Weed
30 Dec. 1994, Woodstock, NY

Editor's Preface

What a surprise to be asked to help bring LUNA YOGA to American audiences. What a bigger surprise to find myself resonating in so many ways with Adelheid Ohlig, to see myself mirrored in her thoughts, her feelings, even her journeys. After all, she is German and I am American, we live in different parts of the globe. Then I realized that it is not so surprising.

Adelheid writes of the importance of menstruation and the need for women to heal and empower themselves. I, too, write about menstruation and lead workshops that empower women. She was led to reclaim her feminine self (after years of denying it while working as a journalist) when she lost her period and contracted cervical cancer. I, too, had to learn to value, honor, and heal my feminine self (after years of success in a very male-defined world) when I began to have debilitating menstrual cramps.

We are all women who have lived our lives within a system that does not value the feminine. Our cycles are not honored or respected, our sexuality is feared and misunderstood. We have spent millennia being shamed, repressed and invalidated for being feminine, to the point where we now, in great numbers, get cancer in our sexual organs, have our breasts cut off (cancer, again), and cannot even access our own deep innate wisdom which is the birthright of women: our inner Wise Woman.

Although the points of connection between Adelheid and myself made the job of editing LUNA YOGA enjoyable, I must admit that this was my most challenging assignment to date as an editor. And now that this is complete and the book is in the reader's hands—where it most definitely should be—I can breathe a deep sigh of relief and joy. Blessings on all your journeys.

Amy Sophia Marashinsky
September, 1994

Why LUNA YOGA?

When I began this book, I asked myself, "Adelheid, is this book really needed?" Isn't there already enough information? Isn't the market flooded with suggestions on movement arts? Do I want to be using lots of paper to make a book? And what can you learn from books anyway?

Despite these truths, I felt compelled to write this book. I did it because human interaction is vitally important to me and I want to share my healing journey with you. I did it because people repeatedly asked me to. I did it so my workshop participants (and those who cannot take a workshop with me) can look up exercises as they wish. I did it so you can read about LUNA YOGA.

I wrote this book hoping to inspire you. If you have some experience in body therapies, I wrote it to stir your curiosity about new ways to combine and use this or that exercise. If you have little or no experience in body therapies, movement, or Yoga, I advise you to be cautious: a book is no substitute for a teacher.

This book can stimulate you and prompt you to further explore for yourself; it will present you with new ideas and introduce you to the subject. But, in order to experience LUNA YOGA to its fullest, it is best to have a teacher, someone who can guide you and encourage you through the rough spots and hard times. This person can observe your practice, and recommend certain postures that best suit your individual life situation. Your teacher can gently remind you to take delight in yourself and in the exercises. Remember, healing doesn't happen when we clench our teeth and do something "because we're supposed to."

For absolute safety, you can go for a medical check-up before you begin your LUNA YOGA program. Do not go beyond the range and limitations of your own body, your own physical endurance. It is absolutely vital that you take delight in the exercises. LUNA YOGA is designed to nourish your joy, awaken your vitality, and make you curious about life. These qualities will then lead you to heal body and soul, spirit and emotions.

Author's Foreword

I am at a point in my life where there is much breakdown, change and transformation. Last night, the borders between East and West Germany were broken down; yesterday, my niece Teresa was transformed by giving birth to her daughter Rosamaria; and about nine months ago my life changed when I signed the contract for this book.

What the opening of Germany's borders means for me is that I, too, can now express myself without boundaries and share the experiences that have influenced me. That the world is now a place where information can pass freely without restrictions, without walls.

Writing this book was similar to a birth, preceded by nine months' gestation. During this time I sifted through knowledge collected in the course of my life, discussed experiences with friends, thought and mused.

The knowledge that I want to pass on was won from breakdowns, changes and transformations, and is transforming itself constantly. I am not introducing a static theory, a rigid set of rules. To the contrary, I want to show exercises, share ideas, and encourage you to discover and explore for yourself.

I put LUNA YOGA before you for discussion—and with that, myself. I want to give guidance and examples and inspire you to think and muse about fertility.

What does our fertility entail? How can we live it and unfold it in all its diversity? Does it not consist of much more than physical fertility, does it not include our entire power to inspire, create and bring forth?

The wealth that I am spreading out here is the combined experience of different people, times, and places. Some of it may strike you as new, other parts may seem very old. I have gathered from diverse cultures and stories all that can enhance fertility.

This book brings together classical Yoga on the one hand and Aviva Steiner's menstrual calisthenics on the other. I want this material to serve as a stepping stone for women and men to experience new ways of promoting vital sexual health. I want to inspire your own creativity and playful exploration of your own vitality, to help you reach a spontaneous expression of your joy and zest for life.

Adelheid Ohlig
November 9, 1989

LUNA YOGA

PART ONE

ROOTS

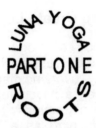

LUNA YOGA
PART ONE
ROOTS

My Story

I will tell you my story:
It is a journey that I had to take.
A journey of discovery
a journey of recovery
a tale woven from the fabric of my being.
This story of mine
could be yours or your sister's
could be hers or her mother's
could be theirs or their grandmother's.
This story of mine is the story
of the Goddess.
For as women, we are all the Goddess
and we have all lived within the confines of the patriarchy
had to remember who we are
awaken our feminine self
take back our female bodies
honor
our cycles
delight in our sexual vitality.
And as women, all women's stories are our story.
This is our story.
May I tell it well
and may it please you all.

How I Came to Create LUNA YOGA

I came to the study of Yoga out of desperation. Desperation, despair and depression. I was in the turmoil of my first year at university, overwhelmed by life and close to suicide, when my brother, a psychologist, recommended I study Yoga. I did and it really saved my life.

In 1978, I started training as a Yoga teacher, while continuing long hours at my high-tech job as an editor for several news agencies.

In the early eighties, I was diagnosed with cervical cancer. Cancer. My mother died of cancer, after numerous operations, radiation treatments and repeated chemotherapy, as did several aunts and uncles. Still, I never imagined in my wildest nightmares that this disease would hit me. After all, I had what I thought was a healthy lifestyle: eating vegetarian nearly all my life, doing my Yoga exercises regularly since I was twenty, meditating almost every day, enjoying my work as a journalist.

No, not me. Others, yes, but not me. And so it happened. I was in my mid-thirties and at my gynecologist's for my yearly exam, when she told me to come back after three months because there were "very suspicious cells" in my cervix. I didn't take this seriously: I went to Japan on assignment, traveled throughout Asia and returned to the doctor a year later. This time the diagnosis was grim. She told me that the cells in my cervix were malignant and that I had a carcinoma in situ. She then began to explain the normal procedure of operation, radiation, and chemotherapy to me, and I burst right into tears.

No, I did not want that. Were there any other options? Her answer was No. It felt like I was handed a death sentence. I left the office, crying.

The next few weeks were spent visiting other doctors,

having PAP smears taken, and hearing the same cervical cancer diagnosis. I thought of my relatives and how they had died horrifically, despite following doctors' orders to operate, radiate, and opiate.

I watched my cat and other animals. What did they do when they were sick? Certainly not go to a hospital. Well, nor would I.

I searched for alternatives and found a general practitioner who was supportive of my ideas on self-healing and promised to help me with prescriptions, even though it was not the normal medical approach. Now I had an ally and I began to have hope. I also found women who had had the same class 5 PAP diagnosis I had, and had chosen routes other than surgery. And they had changed their lives.

As I began to reflect and seriously take stock of my lifestyle, I noticed that in working long hours at my high-tech job, something didn't seem right. I also noticed that my entire life was organized around my job. I probed deeper. I did more Yoga. I meditated and listened and waited. Then I heard it! A small, quiet voice coming from the depths of my being, telling me that although what I was doing in the world was valuable and rewarding, it was no longer really satisfying my inner longings. You see, work was easy, colleagues were friendly, traveling was exciting and stimulating, but I was not content. And if truth be told, I was bored and sometimes depressed. The question now was: What did I want to do? What would bring me happiness and joy?

"Cancer is a very strong signal, it shows that you are bored with life. It is a very tricky and socially acceptable way to commit suicide," one of my friends had the courage to tell me. This was hard for me to swallow, and yet it was true. Living involves choosing. And the choice is about cutting: something will have to be cut and you get to decide. Do you choose the cut in your body (via operation) or in your life (letting go and making changes)?

Empowered by this realization I chose to "cut out" my job. Then I took time for myself. With the help of my friends, I discovered alternative medicine. I received acupuncture, took homeopathic remedies and got massages regularly.

I injected mistletoe extract, went into psychotherapy, and took lessons in breathing and a form of musical healing called sounding. I tried diets and oil massages. I got in touch with my feelings and went through rage, disillusionment, grief, and numbness.

Then I asked myself: Could connecting with my feminine self and getting my cycles back bring about a change in consciousness, a change in lifestyle, that would support and promote a healthy female body? This question assisted me in getting in touch with my fears about being a woman and what that meant.

As I journeyed deep into my fears, what came up for me was anger at the invalidation of the feminine by the patriarchal structure we all live in. If you are a woman then you are not important. Look at the way our cycles are treated: menstruation should be hidden and sanitized, childbirth should be in hospitals and sanitized and menopause should not be experienced at all, for women should be forever young. No honoring or importance. It is no wonder that as I rose to the top of my profession in a male-dominated field, I stopped cycling. I had, in effect, become "the best man for the job."

Still exploring my cycle as a possible answer, I heard about a woman in Israel, Aviva Steiner, who had discovered a series of exercises that could induce menstruation and ovulation. I went to study with her. After studying with Aviva for only a couple of days, I started menstruating for the first time in three years! I felt elated. Elated because I had regained my menstruation, which meant I was regaining my health, and elated because these exercises were what I had been looking for. This was the work that I wanted to do. There was something here that I could explore, something that excited me, something that challenged me. Life was fun again and I felt joyful and happy. I stayed with Aviva, studying with her for several months, and got her permission to teach her exercises. This was the birth of LUNA YOGA.

It was also the disappearance of my carcinoma in situ. Two years had passed since my first class 5 PAP diagnosis. I felt that now was a good time to get another test. The result was a class 1 PAP, a diagnosis of healthy cells. As I had not believed the PAP testing the first time around and had gone for several tests, I had the cells of my cervix tested three times at three different institutes: the results were unanimously class 1 PAP. I had done it! For two years I had trusted my own inner wisdom as it led me to leave my job, experiment with alternative therapies, confront my fears, and learn to honor my feminine self. In the process I had healed and wholed myself. I felt powerful and vibrantly alive.

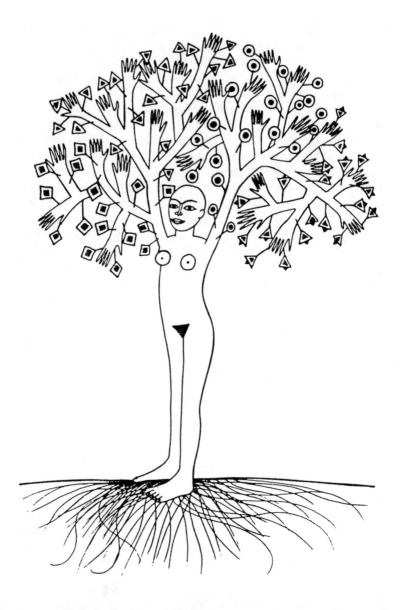

Symbols of LUNA YOGA

The Image

LUNA YOGA to me is like a tree, not a common tree, but a special one. Its roots are in Yoga (which I began studying in 1967). Its trunk is formed by Aviva Steiner's exercises (I have been her apprentice since 1981). The branches and twigs of the tree have grown during my travels around the world and continue to sprout.

I am always looking for dances, rites, movements, affirmations and techniques that in some way influence fertility. I view fertility in its widest sense, as lust for life and joy in one's body (aspects of fertility which are ignored in the western world). The leaves and flowers of this LUNA YOGA tree are the experiences arising from the exercises; the experiences I have, and the experiences you have. And finally, the fruits which ripen are different every time each person practices LUNA YOGA.

The Name

The phrase LUNA YOGA is a joint creation of psychologist Jutta Ruhl-Thomas and myself. We were planning a workshop discussing the idea that menstrual problems are an expression of women's life situations, and we were searching for an attractive title. I am a Yoga teacher; the moon (La Luna) has represented the female since olden times. So it came to us, LUNA YOGA, to connect the changing phases of the moon with the changing moods of our womanly lives, to help us learn to value our changes in a new and positive way.

The Moon

Of course LUNA YOGA has a lot to do with the moon. She grows, becomes full and round, wanes again, and disappears completely. She is moody, fickle, and in constant change. Mood comes from moon. Women are said to be moody, but if we want to be successful in our patriarchal society, we have to put our moods aside and keep smiling.

LUNA YOGA rouses our delight in the changeability of nature, and welcomes the moods of the moon. Our moony moody days bring our lives variety and sprightliness. When we make friends with our changes, we don't become weaker but stronger. We don't need to correct our moods or interfere with them. The moon reminds us to resonate and become whole with all of our moods.

In the symbol of the changing phases of the moon I find an image for my own changing moods and changing body. There is a rhythm to the phases of the moon that noticeably or unnoticeably influences life as well as tides on the earth. This rhythm is an important part of LUNA YOGA: the moon, the tides, the breath, fertility.

Yoga: Unison of Body, Mind, and Spirit
And the Integration into Nature

On the Indian subcontinent, thousands of years ago, wise women and men observed nature, the course of the heavenly bodies, and the cycle of the seasons. They studied the movements of animals and the life of humans. They examined illness and wellness, experimented, tested, and finally arrived at a body of knowledge of ways to promote and protect health and vitality. Their recommendations were collected and summarized in eight levels of Yoga:

Universal Commandments and Guidelines for Self-Discipline (*Yama* and *Niyama* in Sanskrit), Body Postures and Movements (*Asanas*), Breathing Techniques (*Pranayama*), Exercises for the Senses (*Pratyahara*), Concentration Techniques (*Dharana*) and Meditations (*Dhyana*). According to the ancients, following this type of healthy and conscious lifestyle will lead to a state of balance between body, mind, and spirit. You experience a unity with nature, the cosmos, or even the Divine. This state is called *samadhi*.

The word Yoga originates from Sanskrit, an ancient East Indian language, and it means: "to unite, to connect, to combine, to join," as in English "yoke," German "joch." So Yoga means the Union of Body, Mind and Spirit, the Oneness with Ourselves. It unites us with nature and connects us to the divine within.

Pranayama controls and shapes breathing. It is said in Yoga that at our birth we receive a certain number of breaths, and depending on how quickly or slowly we breathe, our life will be short or long.

Through *Pratyahara* we learn the conscious use of our senses. *Dharana* strengthens our ability to concentrate. Meditation — *Dhyana*—helps us to focus and find our center. In *Samadhi* we experience harmony and union.

Asanas promote well-being and its enhancement. In performing the postures, we pay attention, sense, reflect, are present with body and soul. The exercises are done very slowly and consciously. We often pause, hold a specific position, observe our breath, and listen to our own body.

Yoga is not a form of calisthenics in which we technically execute some motions while our thoughts and feelings are wandering about somewhere else. Yoga brings us into total beingness by focusing our awareness on our body and breath. It brings us "home" to ourselves by centering us in our body through our breath.

When we are centered in our body, and can breathe deeply in a relaxed way, we then experience well-being and a quiet, gentle sense of our own power. Yoga, therefore, is a gift that we give ourselves. The centeredness and consciousness of our body that we obtain through the practice of Yoga can also assist us in strengthening our self-healing powers.

Yoga is a way to come from the outside to the inside, from the external to the internal, from the hustle and bustle of life to inner silence, the peace within. Yoga makes us fit. It helps us find our own strength and power by drawing us to our own source of energy. It is a method of curing and healing with movement, breathing exercises and meditation, plus concentration. By concentrating on the movement and coordinating it with our breathing rhythm, we develop body consciousness. We become aware of ourselves, who we really are, and unfold our own inner beauty.

Many traditions were formed within Yoga from the time of its inception, and a diversity of schools developed.

Bhakti Yoga is the yoga of devotion and love. *Janana* Yoga centers around knowledge and the intellect. *Anna* Yoga deals with nutrition, diets, and medicinal plants. *Karma* Yoga is the yoga of action and deeds. *Mantra* Yoga focuses on meditation on a certain sound, a mantra.

Hatha Yoga, the system best known in the west, concentrates on physical exercise. "Ha" is the sun and "Tha" is the moon, thus Hatha Yoga will create a harmony of sun and moon, i.e., bring the male and female energies within us into creative interplay. Some translate Hatha to mean a way of learning to control powerful energies.

Tantra Yoga (also known as Tantric Yoga) is, according to research, the oldest system. Tantra means the "fabric," the web of all life. Its origins are said to date back to 20,000 B.C.E. and stem from Chaldea and Mesopotamia. Many magic rituals which are part of Tantra are still practiced today in Buddhism and Hinduism. Tantra emphasizes the union of man and woman sensually and symbolically. The intention is not only the fusion of woman and man as a couple, but also the interweaving of female and male aspects within ourselves. Carl Gustav Jung described his concepts of Anima and Animus in a similar way.

Rajah Yoga is the royal path and integrates different aspects of the other schools.

Yoga is a very old philosophy and healing art. It was already well developed on the Indian subcontinent 6000 years ago. Documents found in the Indus Valley showing figures in different Yoga positions date back to 3000 years ago. Figures of rock and clay, dated at 6000 years old, showing individuals in Yoga positions are frequently found. These sculptures portray both women and men. In some areas more female than male figures have been found, indicating that the origins of Yoga may have been feminine. And here I would like to state that with its strong support and balancing of the endocrine system, Yoga might have been part of the flowering of the Goddess-oriented matrifocal culture.

Today, Yoga focusing on women is hard to find. Yoga is inherently a holistic science and, of course, includes both women and men. Notice how in Indian mythology there is always a couple: the goddess and the god, and one cannot do without the other. Shiva, the male dormant power, needs Shakti, the female creative energy, to create the world. Creation itself can be seen as a process of ever-changing merging of male and female qualities.

However, Yoga has become man's domain. Women's knowledge of it has become veiled. When you find the sentence in the Yoga books, "This is not for women," or if your Yoga teacher tells you so, you can be sure that, in fact, this is a special exercise/movement for women. Many Yoga books write absurdities about menstruation, mostly from the male viewpoint. In LUNA YOGA women's cycles are dealt with from the woman's perspective.

Yoga goes beyond the unity of body, mind, and spirit. Nothing happens in a void; we live in a community that includes not only other people, but other living beings, and even the so-called inanimate world, nature, the whole cosmos. All of this is considered and integrated in Yoga.

Yoga is timely. In an ecological sense, Yoga helps us make use of all our experiences and integrate and accept them without judgment. As we develop attention through our yoga practice we learn to observe calmly and perceive the reactions of our body, our feelings and thoughts. Thus, an increasingly clearer image of our own state of being can emerge. For example, instead of fighting against discomfort, we allow it in and go through it. When we resist or fight against any feeling we have, it doesn't go away. We just end up depleting our vital energy. When we open to what we are feeling, the feeling transforms and we find ourselves with greater energy and greater health.

From East India and the origins of Yoga—where our LUNA YOGA tree is rooted—our journey now leads us to Israel, where Aviva Steiner made some incredible discoveries about women. These discoveries form the trunk of LUNA YOGA.

Aviva Steiner and Her Discoveries

Aviva Steiner was born in Hungary in 1930. She emigrated to Israel when she was a young woman. There she embarked on a career as a dancer. She studied with Gertrude Kraus, and performed in kibbutzim theater and opera. She spent four years as a classical ballerina and seven years as a jazz dancer. Then she ended her dance career and trained as a physical therapist and as a Yoga teacher. The new focus of her work was physiotherapy and various other body therapies. Her training in anatomy stimulated many questions.

If someone can wiggle their ears, why not also move their internal muscles? If yogis and yoginis (men and women practicing Yoga) can control their heart beat and the functions of their internal organs, why couldn't women influence their menstruation and ovulation and be able to regulate their fertility?

Wanting to regulate her own fertility, Aviva began to seek answers to her questions. She studied anatomy books and familiarized herself with the female body and its possibilities. She became an acute observer of her own physical movement and kept track of it on a daily basis while also studying the body's functions. She closely explored her own cycle.

At that time, she taught gymnastics, dance, and Yoga in different institutions in Israel. After several months of teaching movement in a retirement home, several older women came to her and proudly reported: "I'm bleeding again!"

At first, Aviva was shocked, but then realized that here was an opportunity to find out to what extent ovulation and menstruation could be influenced through movement.

Aviva set aside time for experimentation. She compared her cycles with those of her women friends. Together, they observed how their physical activities affected their periods. Based on this exchange of experiences, Aviva Steiner developed a specific system of movements for female reproductive health. Only after a decade of research did she make her findings public at a conference in Tel Aviv in 1974.

The topic of the conference was sexual medicine. Questions were posed about natural birth control. Aviva reported on her experiences with gymnastics and dance. She said that certain types of specific exercises practiced at certain times and for certain durations can either promote or decrease fertility. Shocked silence greeted her findings. In amazement, the medical doctors learned how physical exercise can influence such highly complicated processes as menstruation and ovulation.

Today it is no secret that athletes often don't ovulate. Anorexic women, who combine deficient diets with obsessive physical exercise regimes, also lose their periods. The same goes for female body builders. Even exercises like aerobics, stretching, and jogging can disturb the female rhythm if done excessively.

Aviva Steiner continued to improve her exercises as she continued to observe diverse forms of human and animal movement. Her system got more and more complex. Finally, she published a booklet titled *Physical Exercises as a Solution for Menstrual Cycle and Pregnancy—A Series of Exercises Which Cause the Onset of Menses According to the Desire of Women* (original title in Hebrew). Then she registered her system with the World Health Organization in Geneva and with the International Patent Bureau. She received a copyright from the National Council for Research and Development in Tel Aviv and registered her exercises with the Population Crisis Committee in Washington, D.C.

Aviva discovered that a woman's energy source is in her pelvis, in her sexual organs. If a woman's energy is allowed to flow freely from her sexual organs into the rest of her body, the woman will live a healthy, long life and have tremendous energy and vitality. If the energy is locked in the pelvis, reproductive problems and a variety of diseases from PMS to cancer are promoted.

The pelvises of most, if not all, of the women I meet are immobile. It is considered "whorish" in our patriarchal Judeo-Christian society for women to walk with their hips freely flowing. They are looked down upon and the movement is described as "unlady-like" or "done just to excite men." In reality, in order to walk and circulate the energy through the body, the pelvis/hip area has to move. In our culture women are allowed to breathe into their pelvis only when giving birth. Strong pelvic thrusts in dances are considered obscene, and the fact that this may even awaken pleasure and sexual desire seems indecent to some.

I believe this lack of connection to our wombs and sexual organs is the cause of our menstrual/menopausal/infertility problems. The energy in our pelvis is locked and blocked by society so we find it hard to be pleased with or receive pleasure from our genitals. This is why Steiner's system was a revelation to me: it opened up my pelvis for the first time in my life.

Aviva taught me to breathe into my sexual organs, she gave me permission—in fact, she demanded—that I move my pelvis, slowly, sensually, vigorously. All the so-called "forbidden" ways. What I discovered was that the freeing of my pelvis increased my vitality and my sexual pleasure!

East India and Israel. Yoga and Aviva Steiner's exercises—they form the roots and trunk of LUNA YOGA. But what, you may ask, is the whole of LUNA YOGA?

Women's Blood Mysteries

In matrifocal cultures, women are honored and seen as the Goddess. The power of their fertility, both to give birth and to green the Earth, as evidenced in their ability to menstruate, is respected and held sacred. Menstrual blood has been used through the ages as an Earth fertilizer *par excellence*. During planting season, women would plant the seeds and then fertilize the ground with their menstrual blood. The menstrual cycle is seen as creatively powerful, giving birth not only to children but all nourishment.

During the time of bleeding women's ability to dream, have visions and attain altered states of consciousness is strong. When moontime visions are sought, answers come, whether of pottery patterns, or the location of herds of food animals, or solutions to social problems.

For thousands of years the blood mysteries of women were an important part of the life of most human societies. The rituals that women create for their own well-being, to protect and nurture their extreme psychic sensitivity and power during menstruation and menopause, childbirth and puberty, serve all of society, not only the individual woman. About 5000 years ago, this changed in many places, most notably Europe. There, matrifocal wisdom has been repressed, and the special menstrual/menopausal/fertility rituals that once nourished all have been calcified into rules and taboos and used to create shame that separates women from their own power and the power of the blood mysteries.

Today, many doctors and researchers see the menstrual cycle as unnecessary. Though some scientists theorize that there may be a relationship between the higher life expectancy of women and our reproductive cycles (because we constantly renew our organism through menstruation), some view women's monthly bleeding as decadent.

A naturopath, for instance, states that if women were to eat raw foods exclusively, they wouldn't need this "purification process," and G. Breuer, a medical doctor, asks in a German journal of natural science (*Naturwissenschaftliche Rundschau*, October, 1981), *Is Menstruation Contrary to Nature*? The gynecologist Fritz Beller writes in the German magazine *Die Zeit* (issue 6, 1985), "I consider attempts to prevent menstruation completely as meaningful, because I believe that the monthly cycle is one of the few errors of nature."

And women, too, come to think of their powerful bleeding time as an error, if for no other reason than that they are "irregular"—that is, they don't menstruate every 28 days. But studies done in the United States, Australia, Great Britain and France show only 18 to 27 percent of all women of child-bearing age having a "regular period" every 28 days. About three-quarters of all women have their own individual cycles with varying lengths between periods and fluctuating durations of the periods. When a standard is applied to something as individual and personally unique as the menstrual cycle, then women's health suffers, as in the notion that 75 percent of women menstruate irregularly.

Repression of women's menstrual power *literally* hurts women. Experts in women's health care, such as Christiane Northrup, M.D. and Susun Weed, say that the overwhelming majority of reproductive/menstrual/menopausal problems are a direct result of patriarchal disempowerment of women's mysteries.

A study done on the influence of religion on women's menstrual well-being showed that women who were most likely to suffer from menstrual pain and problems were the ones whose religion told them they were unclean or that they had to be submissive to men. (In one religion women are denied communion when having their period.) Women with the smallest percentage of menstrual problems belonged to churches where women can become priests or even bishops.

Then there are the conscious or unconscious messages from our mothers or other females in our environment. How did we experience our menarche, the first blood? What examples of the menstrual cycle did we experience as we were growing up? Were we taught that the fluctuations of our bodies make us more adaptable and resistant? Or were we told we had the "curse." No wonder we feel conflict about our cycles and try to deny our very beingness as women.

Women's menstrual and reproductive problems often begin during periods of stress. One cause of the stress is the conflict of being female in a male-oriented, male-dominated society where there are few positive views of the feminine and little support of the female cycle. In many cultures women are highly revered, but also avoided because of their relationship to blood, which is seen as a symbol for life and death. In the past, blood mysteries were seen as the divine power of women; they formed the basis of religious rites which we enact even today in some cultures. The power of woman—say the Native Americans—lies in her ability to give life and to use this creativity in different ways. Patriarchal societies, however, view women's blood mysteries as a threat to their power, and have suppressed women and their knowledge of their menstrual power.

In modern civilization the discrimination against women and their cycles manifests in many different ways. In the United States, for example, there are very few companies that offer fully paid maternity leave (sometimes classified as "disability leave"), and no workplaces that give time off for the menstrual cycle. The message we are given via the media and in the workplace is that we are to keep our cycles hidden (as in the tampon commercials) so we can be like men (who don't bleed). Of course our bodies express such conflict and this disturbed relationship manifests in disharmonies of our uterus, ovaries, menses, fertility.

Modern advertising, with its arsenal of youth, beauty, and money, dictates that menstruation should not be seen or heard, felt or smelled. Women should perceive or display nothing of their physical changes. The days of the period should be like any other day. Tampons have applicators so women don't have to touch or contaminate themselves "down there." Nobody should notice that women have cycles. Everything should run smoothly. When it doesn't, take painkillers, use suppositories. Science, too, is used to promoting the latest in menstrual aversion, whether it's in helping women hide those "unpleasant facts of life"—like hot flashes and premenstrual tension—or in telling us that careers cause infertility.

Can we change? During the 1970s many of the newly founded women's collectives in Europe included in their bylaws a provision for each woman to take off one day a month for menstruation. Only a few women claimed this benefit. Some considered the free menstrual day as uneconomical. Others viewed it as a reduction of their femininity. Twenty years later, women's collectives in Europe consider this day— once celebrated as revolutionary—as a mere historical curiosity.

The power of menstruation is still honored in many cultures, in ways wondrous, amazing, and inspiring. There are many Native American nations where the women's cycles are considered a source of power for the woman; where women are revered for their ability to bleed and to give birth; where they are honored for their ability to give life, but also allowed to refuse this role. Women past menopause are the guardians of tradition, and wisdom is attributed to them. (According to many ethnologists, rites of circumcision for men in different cultures are an imitation of the female cycle.)

In Sri Lankra, the entire family celebrates with a huge feast when a girl has her first blood. She wears red clothing, which symbolizes joy.

Many rules and taboos about menstruation, that today appear discriminating, were originally rituals created by women for their own well-being.

In ancient Japan, menstrual huts for women were situated in the most beautiful places: along the seashore, often on top of a hill. There the women could withdraw to spend time in solitude, or retreat with others.

In most rural communities a woman's menstrual blood is known to be a powerful fertilizer. At special times women give their blood to the earth to insure the fertility of the fields and an abundant harvest.

In Southeastern India, among still-existent matriarchal tribes, women move to the ocean to meditate during their menses. Their retreat, their time of self communion, is honored as a service to the community. Their clothes are washed and all their chores are done by the male members of the tribe while they menstruate. When, after a few days, the women return to the village, they are full of inner strength. They are welcomed back by their men and pampered with their favorite foods.

Among the Shasta Indians of northern California, a girl at her menarche goes into a special menstrual hut that has been prepared for her and remains there for about ten days. She is accompanied by her mother or an older woman who takes care of her, bathing her, caring for her, feeding her. Everything she dreams while she is here will come true.

Can we change? Can we redream the blood mysteries? Yes! I've done it. So have other women. We do LUNA YOGA, to begin sensing into our bellies. As our memories surface, we acknowledge our menstrual experiences. If there is anger at what we experienced menstrually, we give that rage its voice, then agree to let it go. Once we do that, we begin to create our menstrual experience as nurturing, joyful, supportive, whatever we need it to be for ourselves. We can let it connect us with the Grandmothers, with Earth Mother, with the Moon, with the Goddess and with our Feminine Self. We become one with the great spiral of all women and we become whole/ healthy.

A Special Note To Men

Men in our western cultures need to know LUNA YOGA, for when we all live freely together or want to create new forms of living together, then mutual respect is an important precondition. Thus, menstruation and menopause, contraception and creation, are also subjects for men: if they live with women, it simply is a part of it. New understanding of one another can grow from it.

In matriarchal Native American cultures women don't rule over men, but both carry responsibilities for different domains of life. Women and men have their own rituals to strengthen their personal powers, and joint rites to benefit the society. Thus men and women meet as persons of equal value and equal power.

I am writing mostly about women, because I am one and because I work with women. Nonetheless, I believe that what is said here has relevance for men as well. We want to live together in new ways and not congeal into conventions that have become useless. Thus I want to present LUNA YOGA not as a pruned ornamental shrub, but as a growing, changing tree, as the Turkish poet Nazim Hikmet has described it:

> To live
> single and free
> like a tree
> and brotherly like a forest
> is our desire.

And sisterly it works just as well.

LUNA YOGA

PART TWO

USING LUNA YOGA

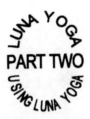

What Is LUNA YOGA?

LUNA YOGA is the touch of a moonbeam on your skin, a gentle awakening to pleasure that can be felt in your own body.

LUNA YOGA increases your energy and vitality by supporting and encouraging you to breathe into your sexual organs and shake, rattle and roll your pelvis.

LUNA YOGA is a dance of joy and zest, a dance of life.

LUNA YOGA is a path to reclaiming yourself as Woman.

LUNA YOGA is a joyful way to energy and sexual vitality.

LUNA YOGA is the combination of Yoga's ancient matriarchal roots (and postures too long denied to women), Aviva Steiner's menstrual calisthenics, and fertility dances that I encountered on my travels.

LUNA YOGA takes its name "Luna" from the moon, the symbol of the feminine, the unconscious, the intuitive. In ancient times women's cycles were aligned with the moon: ovulation was at the full moon and bleeding during the dark of the moon. The moon and her cycles were considered a visible representation of the Triple Goddess: the crescent moon was the Maiden, the full moon was the Mother, and the dark of the moon, the Crone. The dark of the moon was also referred to as the time of endings, the time of rebirth, and the time when the moon renewed herself to begin her cycle's dance afresh. Therefore, LUNA YOGA is the woman's way of connecting to body, mind and spirit, invented *by* women *for* women.

LUNA YOGA unlocks immense vitality, our birthright as women because the exercises focus on our sexual organs, the home of our life force. LUNA YOGA is a wakeup call to our sleeping sexuality, heightening sexual pleasure through the use of breath and specific muscle strengthening exercises. (Most ancient cultures honored sex as important for well-being, health and wholeness.)

How Does LUNA YOGA Work?

LUNA YOGA works by enhancing self-healing powers.

LUNA YOGA works by embracing and nourishing the whole. LUNA YOGA works by being fun.

LUNA YOGA works by means of gentle sensing exercises.

These are done slowly and in time with the rhythm of your own breath. They allow you to develop a sense of your own body. You not only discover muscle and tendon movement, but little by little, experience the deeper layers of your body. You develop a sense of your inner organs. By breathing more fully into the deeper layers of your body, you can increase or decrease your circulation and bring warmth into your body.

LUNA YOGA works by means of breath. Breath, which connects us with held feelings. Muscle tissues hold feelings. Breath moves them, bringing them to consciousness. When feelings emerge—how shall we name them? Often we think of words with negative connotations when we experience new bodily sensations: we say that we have aches and pains, hurts and so forth. But maybe it is not pain; maybe it is just the first time we *feel* something in some part of our body. Be inventive with language; try out new words to express new perceptions. Instead of fearing your feelings or suppressing them, give yourself permission to feel, no matter what you call the feeling, and let your feelings flow.

During the breathing exercises we notice where there is tension. Since describing something in negative terms can lock us into feeling negative, I'd like to invite you to see what is happening that is your ally, is there for your benefit. When you name something as being there for your benefit, it becomes just that. Let the tension remind you to breathe deeper and slower. And again and again become aware of how you breathe and which sensations go along with it. This attentive breathing will not only improve the oxygen supply in your lungs, but in your entire body, in each single cell, and your metabolism will be vitalized.

LUNA YOGA trains us to focus on our breathing and how we feel. This attentive breathing will not only improve the oxygen supply to our lungs, but to our entire body. In each single cell metabolism becomes more energetic, more joyous.

LUNA YOGA works by means of powerful fertility dances that vibrate our tissues, circulate energy and revive our body, mind, and spirit.

LUNA YOGA works by supplying oxygen and nutrients to the pelvic organs, increasing elimination of old cells and unneeded hormones, and increasing utilization of new energy.

LUNA YOGA works by stimulating and tonifying the endocrine system. With great probability, due to the intensive concentration on our sexual organs, a feedback cycle is formed with the pituitary gland which directs our entire endocrine system. The gentle sensing exercises, the focusing of our breath on the sexual organs, and the dances all help to regulate our hormones.

LUNA YOGA works by gently stretching and twisting the back, making our spinal muscles stronger and more flexible. Muscle tensions, which often pinch the spinal nerves as they exit the vertebral column, are relaxed. The entire nervous system becomes well supplied with blood due to increased circulation, which also creates greater warmth. It is possible that at first, LUNA YOGA may bring up old buried pains. They will, after a period of adjustment, eventually disappear, and an enhanced sense of well-being will spread out over your entire body. You will experience vitality, pleasure, and creativity on all levels.

LUNA YOGA works with the help of herbal wisdom and Wise Woman Ways from my home state of Hessia, to nourish, calm and tonify. Herbal baths and oils with healing and harmonizing effects act on our sense organs. Meditations bring us into our own center and visualizations help us prepare our new outer reality, harness our imagination and create the best possible reality for ourselves.

Here's how LUNA YOGA works for me: I have discovered, after watching the patterns in my own life, that illness doesn't strike me out of the blue. When I take on too many things to do and don't give myself enough nurturance or rest, I get sick. Illness reminds me to pay attention to my needs. After all, if I am unable to give to myself, how can I expect to be able to give to others?

I've discovered that change is easier when I recognize the patterns in my life that don't serve me joyfully. Then I can name them, and if I wish, I can transform them. Do I hold onto my misery and my need to feel bad? Or do I allow myself to feel my feelings and let them transform? Energy is where I put it. Do I spend adequate time in my feelings? Do I wallow in despair as a way of invalidating myself or hiding from joy?

LUNA YOGA works by nourishing our ability to choose what brings energy, vitality and joy to ourselves, to women.

LUNA YOGA works by combining a system of breathing with joyful physical exercises designed specifically for the well-being of women and their reproductive cycles.

Here's how LUNA YOGA works: a group of eight women met over a period of several months, once a week, to practice LUNA YOGA and talk about their cycles. The results were profound. Women with intense menstrual cramping experienced less painful periods. A few women with anorexic tendencies, who had ceased menstruating, began menstruating again. One woman, who was locked for years in a pitched battle with her cycle, was able to make peace with it. This influenced her fertility and she was able to realize her dream and become pregnant.

LUNA YOGA works by nourishing body and mind with variety. All our senses want expression and need material and spiritual nourishment. It feels good to experiment with different physical movement. Just as we need to eat and sleep, our body needs to move. Unfortunately, we learned at an early age in school to "sit still and keep quiet." And, from force of habit, we continue to do that. One of the most exciting discoveries of my healing journey was finding my body through vigorous physical movement. Aviva encouraged me to shout, to stamp, to make noise, to make my presence felt, to take up space. It was energizing and freeing and ultimately healing.

LUNA YOGA doesn't work as a miracle cure. LUNA YOGA works when body, mind, and spirit want to change. It is important to have illness diagnosed and to have skilled assistance and medical advice while deciding on your course of healing. LUNA YOGA can be a wonderful adjunct to any standard medical treatment. It strengthens the self-healing powers, awakens joy of life, and often brings undreamed of energies.

What Can LUNA YOGA Do?

Both Aviva Steiner and I have observed and experienced these results from regular LUNA YOGA practice:
- Ovulation as well as menstruation can be stimulated.
- The ability to conceive can be improved.
- Implantation of a fertilized egg can be hindered.
- The muscles of the pelvic floor, the uterus (which also is a muscle), and the connective tissue will be strengthened by LUNA YOGA. This is especially important for women who habitually miscarry.
- Cysts and uterine fibroids shrink or disappear.
- Precancerous cells decrease.
- Pain and cramps before and during menses are relieved.
- Endometriosis can be reduced.
- Premenstrual tension can be resolved.
- The entire cycle is harmonized.
- Menopausal symptoms are relieved or don't develop.
- Skin functions improve (pH value, resistance, and moisture of mucous membranes).
- The vicious cycle of bulimia and anorexia ends.
- For men, LUNA YOGA can help to improve the quality and quantity of sperm. Couples may realize their desire for a child, or may discover a different form of fertility: creativity, joy in their work, a change of profession, new levels of partnership, and more.
- Both men and women deepen their delight in sexuality. Some women have reached orgasm for the first time after practicing LUNA YOGA.
- LUNA YOGA connects us with our own inner Wise Woman, our inner ally, who helps us to heal/whole/holy ourselves.

Being Well and Being Ill

My idea of becoming healthy takes the whole person into account. Wellness and illness are but two poles of our lives. Health is not the absence of disease and maybe not even what the World Health Organization has defined it as—a state of total physical, mental, and psychological well-being.

I believe that we are created perfect, exactly as we are. We are equipped with self healing powers (as are other living beings). We need to acknowledge and nourish these powers if we wish to enjoy health and vitality.

Native American medicine women whom I have encountered in my travels describe healing as "the path of beauty." They view illness as a chance to awaken the powers of beauty. They say their cultures seek to reintegrate what has been split off through illness, rather than widening the split by "curing the disease."

In ancient China physicians supposedly were paid for keeping people healthy. Today we pay for our diseases—not just singly, and not just economically for society as a whole pays a dear price emotionally and psychically for the current state of dis-ease.

When we learn to understand illness as a message that lets us know that we need to listen to ourselves more closely, that something needs attention, then we will hear the song of health. Illness is a great teacher, a great ally. To allow ourselves the freedom to be ill and to listen to what that is saying to us is one of the greatest gifts we can give ourselves. Many healers have walked this path: illness as teacher. Some of the gifts that illness gave me were respect for that which nourishes my connection with myself, my connection with the Goddess, and my connection with my inner Wise Woman.

One of the most dehumanizing effects of the industrial revolution is the view of the human body as a machine. One of the miracles of today's medicine is that you now can have replacement parts for those that are injured, malformed, or wear out in your body, just like a machine. Standards work with machines, but it is contrary to human nature to fit to a standard of what's "normal." This is especially true when that standard is based solely on tests done on males. In our medical textbooks and especially in the minds of most medical doctors, naturopaths, and members of other health professions, there is an image of health defined by standards that don't honor the uniqueness of each individual.

If we leave standards aside, we will discover our own form of health. If we put rigid rules away, changeable liveliness will emerge. When we free ourselves from rules and dogmas about our being, then the breezes, winds, storms, hurricanes, typhoons, and whirlwinds of freedom will rage around us, and we will find ourselves daring to choose our own way. Definitions and judgments often hinder us from perceiving what really is. Realization awaits us only in what is—not in what we imagine. Concepts stand in the way, they injure our free view, our open perspective. To take the freedom to be ill and to watch what's being signaled—who would dare that?

A lot would change. We would become a more humane to our selves and each other as we came to recognize our humanness—that which makes us alive—with all its ups and downs, irregularities and abnormalities. Can we dare to live our lives without painting over our different conditions and sacrificing for the sake of uniformity? If we can let ourselves be, and that means to accept how we feel at the present moment, then we can experience ourselves anew and can also let others be and truly tolerate them.

Considering myself as a machine, trying to fit the standard—which in the west is a white, Aryan young male from the middle or upper class—and not paying attention to my femaleness, was a major factor leading to my illness. The diagnosis of cancer began my journey of healing, a journey of discovery of who I was, what I wanted and what I needed in order to live joyfully. On that journey, I learned to let myself be, let myself feel. This was deeply healing. I learned that I was disconnected from my body and that, to heal, I had to find that which really connected me with my body. Through that connection, I learned to be present and feel comfortable in my body.

When I recognized that I was *not* a continuously-functioning machine, I felt my humanness, my body, at last. When we stop comparing and measuring, we arrive at our own well-being. For example, when I was in Japan my blood pressure (90/60) was considered totally normal, while in Germany it is considered low blood pressure. I felt well there and here, too, even if the physicians here expect me to feel tired, without energy, and to have a hard time getting up. The opposite is true.

Have you noticed that the language of Western medicine is a martial one? Enemies are fought against! Diseases are wiped out! Bacteria and germs are overthrown! Surgeons sever and cut out what is considered unnecessary. Women are being asked in their early thirites if they still "need" their uterus, i.e., do they still want to have children. Woman is reduced to a baby machine, female organs reduced to their functions. If a woman doesn't want more children, the unnecessary organs can be removed. In Germany 35 percent of women over 60 have had a total hysterectomy (uterus and ovaries removed). Often the procedure is declared "cancer preventative" surgery.

I don't condemn western medicine: it has given me a number of blessings. But too often it poses as the only possible viewpoint with all other possibilities of healing excluded.

Is natural medicine an alternative? Western medicine looks at the human body as a machine that can be fixed and natural medicine often presents humans as filthy temples that have a need for constant cleansing. The methods used are emesis, colonics, cupping, bloodletting, leeches, fasting and purging. Although the body is viewed as the temple of the soul, if it is constantly necessary to cleanse it and cast out the dung, as if it were a pigsty, then this looks more like body hatred. In homeopathy there are typical remedies for the "nagging crone," the "weepy widow," or the "fickle virgin." There are remedies for indecisive girls or for frigidity. Male analogies are lacking, but the so-called male remedies have attributes with positive connotations. The male remedies are for managers, for movers and shakers, for energetic daredevils, fearless fellows, and similar types.

The Aschner handbook *—The Naturopathic Bible—still recommends applying leeches to the labia if a woman's period is late. Of course, according to the author, such methods are not to be applied to the male genitals.

There's another way. A way where I'm not a machine and not unclean. A way where I don't have to be sick in order to rest and relax. A way where I give myself permission to listen to the messages from my body and not to statements from authorities. When I utilize the different opportunities that life presents to me and I come into wholeness with my feminine self and into harmony with nature, then I will attain health. I want to resonate with the ups and downs of life, the changes of the moon, the cycle of birth, fullness and death, so that I can comprehend health as described by Moshe Feldenkrais, the founder of the body therapy of the same name: "A healthy person is one who can fully live their hidden dreams."

* B. Aschner, *Technik der Konstitutionstherapie* (Technique of Constitutional Therapy), (referred to as "Aschnerbibel"), published by Karl Haug Verlag, Ulm/Donau, 1984, sixth ed.

LUNA YOGA Stories of Healing

Astrid, 17, a student, had "hellish" pains during her menstruation. She came to me hoping that LUNA YOGA would end her intense cramping and that she would recover from her fear of her period. I recommended a specific series of exercises, done with regularity and commitment. Although Astrid felt concerned about her ability to maintain a regular practice, she committed to the program and "threw herself" into those exercises that were especially fun for her. She waited for her next period. It came and went painlessly. She was delighted. Today Astrid practices off and on. Her menses continue almost completely painlessly.

Eva, 20, lives in a communal living arrangement. She doesn't know yet what she wants to do after her high school graduation. She is bulimic and anorexic. Eva wants to break out of the vicious cycle of bingeing and purging and regain her period. She has not cycled in over two years. After a weekend workshop of fairly basic exercises, she set aside half an hour a day for LUNA YOGA. After three months she is bleeding again. She slowly makes friends with food, in her own way, and comes to the conclusion that living in a female body and having a few curves is "quite nice."

Inga, 29, wants to get her high school diploma. She has PMS and feels tired and fatigued for days before her period. Her LUNA YOGA practice helps her to relax. The breathing techniques reduce her premenstrual tension. She is learning to give her self the rest and nurturance she needs at that time of the month.

Olga is in her mid-thirties and suffers from uterine fibroids. Strong menstrual cramps interfere with her ability to work. Her physicians recommend a hysterectomy. Olga came to me eager to try alternative solutions. After a few weeks of daily LUNA YOGA exercises, her pains have lessened. The doctors say the fibroids "appear" to have shrunk.

I met Myriam, a forty-year-old school psychologist, while teaching in Australia. Myriam has a full, completely booked schedule. Each day there is a different exercise program or cultural event. She and Uri, her companion, decided they want to have a child. They have come to me to learn LUNA YOGA because they have been trying to get pregnant and haven't been able to. At the first lesson, I wonder if there is any time and space in their busy schedules for a child, let alone time for love, but I say nothing. At the second session, Myriam has given up Tuesday's jogging. When I come for the third time, Thursday afternoon's bridge game is gone. At the fourth session, Uri and Myriam have decided to take more time for creating spontaneous common activities. Fifth appointment: Myriam waits for her period. Upon my return to Europe I get the news that she is pregnant.

Uma, in her forties, professionally successful, experiences her first menopausal symptoms. She doesn't want hormone replacement therapy, and starts LUNA YOGA. Her hot flashes ease off, and she feels lighter, more serene, and at ease. She likes that she can do her exercises as she pleases and doesn't have to perform a "strict program."

Elisabeth, 63, is told she has cancer and faces a total hysterectomy. Rather than rushing into surgery, she gives herself six months of LUNA YOGA and alternative therapies. When she goes back for her next checkup, her gynecologist is stunned: no precancerous cells are found in her PAP smear. Elisabeth is overjoyed. Her doctor is baffled.

Georgia, a gifted flutist, and her husband, a talented pianist, are in their thirties and have been wanting a child for a long time. But Georgia has very irregular ovulations and she is too heavy as well, and Leonardo's sperm count shows only few fully mature, living sperm. They start LUNA YOGA, and fully enjoy the exercises and joint dances. They put together a daily exercise program of twenty minutes, and once a month, they take four days to do one hour of LUNA YOGA per day.

They choose the mid-cycle days to induce ovulation. Four months later, Leonardo feels stronger and more flexible. His sperm count shows significantly better results. Georgia is thinner and pregnant;

Seventy-seven-year-old Pascale complains of dry, itchy skin and sensitive mucous membranes. She likes LUNA YOGA right away, and feels "on top of the world" with her tailored training series of gentle sensing exercises and harmonizing breathing techniques. The itching disappears. She feels refreshed and her mucous membranes regain their moisture.

In Canada, an entire communal household is devoted to LUNA YOGA. Women and men alike have taken great delight in it and meet on and off for an evening of LUNA YOGA.

In Switzerland, I conducted a LUNA YOGA group that dealt intensively with the subject of menstrual problems. For several months eight women met regularly once a week to practice LUNA YOGA and talk about their cycles. A lot was being activated: the women supported each other to better understand their respective situations, processes of consciousness were initiated, and resistance could be dissolved. This all happened not by way of curing symptoms, but through insights that were gained through body, mind, and spirit. A few women with anorexic tendencies, who had long been without a cycle, started bleeding again. One woman realized her strong fantasy to become pregnant. The interplay of the outer and the inner, the combination of sharing, physical exercises, breathing techniques, and creative activities was a lot of fun. A new understanding for processes in one's own body was awakened, that in turn gave more security to the women to seek out their own paths, even if they were contrary to conventional stereotypes of female behavior. And, yes, these women who had been having many menstrual problems began to experience much less painful periods.

LUNA YOGA

PART THREE

EXERCISES

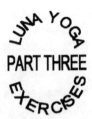

Your LUNA YOGA Practice

LUNA YOGA should be practiced with ease and pleasure on the one hand and with attention and awareness on the other. How can you find the right balance? Probably the book itself will not be sufficient for this. Just to start it out of a gut feeling may not be right for everybody. Therefore I advise you to seek out a teacher and have them explain and demonstrate the basics. (See Resources, page 188) Then you can practice the exercises in your own home. I also advise you to precede your training program with a medical checkup, so you can start at the level appropriate for your capacity.

LUNA YOGA should be fun, and at the same time it requires discipline. If we want to reach a goal, we have to invest energy, but overall we will increase our energy, because training that requires strength brings it back to us. On a long-term basis LUNA YOGA will help us be more awake, lighter, clearer, more joyous.

Therefore it is important to practice the exercises with a sense of the unity of body, mind, and spirit. Don't blindly follow instructions, but perceive your own boundaries. The illustrations in this book are just images. For every person who practices LUNA YOGA, each single exercise can turn out differently. Our physical builds and our flexibility are very diverse.

LUNA YOGA is recreated anew with every person doing it. The LUNA YOGA tree is constantly growing, flowering, and fruiting with myriad forms of beauty as individual and diverse as the people practicing and inevitably changing it. I do not wish to create a rigid structure that confines you, but offer you a way of connecting with your own inner vitality, creativity, and health.

LUNA YOGA, as we have seen, is composed of various elements. Here are specific exercises for each of the aspects of LUNA YOGA: relaxation, breathing, gentle sensing exercises, fertility dances, and pressure point massage.

Relaxation

Relaxation is vital to the LUNA YOGA process. It is the dynamic opposite of tension. Relaxation not only helps us loosen tight muscles, it helps us to let go of preceding events and to engage in the present. Thus, we begin and end our LUNA YOGA sessions with relaxation.

When we relax, we can more easily let go of what was and allow what will be. During relaxation we can feel where our body makes contact with the ground and how we experience this. How do the different parts of our body feel? How does gravity affect us? To what extent are we able to let go of our surroundings and focus inwardly? What is our primary body sensation? What sentiments and images emerge? What is old and what is new? What do we like and dislike? Try not to judge, just simply perceive.

While doing the following relaxations, consciously relax every part of your body while silently thinking of each part: head, shoulders, arms, hands, chest, pelvis, legs, feet. When you begin with your head and cover your entire body with affirmations to relax, ending at the feet, you ground yourself and let go of being too much in your head. Toes, feet, calves, knees, thighs, pelvis, chest, fingers, hands, wrists, elbows, arms, shoulders, head: when you start at the feet and wander upwards to the head, covering the entire body with affirmations of relaxation, you can free yourself from too much gravity.

Coordinate your relaxation with your breath for maximum effectiveness. With every exhalation, let go more and more. Let go of the carbon dioxide you no longer need; exhale from every cell. Let go of all your thoughts and plans and anything that stresses you. Let go of everything that you don't need any more. I don't mean that you ought to suppress anything, but that now you should give yourself over to focusing completely on yourself, your breath, your belly, without tension, without thought, without fear. With every inhalation open more and more. Open to receive fresh oxygen in every cell. Open to receive fresh insights. Open to healing. Open to the deep sense of freedom and power that LUNA YOGA brings.

In deep relaxation, we totally relinquish our selves to our breath while remaining completely conscious. We get involved with ourselves. We discover new and hidden energies in this state of silent self communion. We allow ourselves just to be, without the need to act. We are completely who we are. We renew, and regenerate, and allow the healing energies of the universe to permeate us completely. We feel the unison of body, mind, and spirit and our connection to nature and the universe, and to the divine in each and every thing. We dive deeply into our sensory awareness and we feel and fill every cell of our body with vitality.

A beginning relaxation prepares body and mind to work together with breath and helps us learn to focus on the pelvis. Don't worry about time; let it last as long as you need it to, until you are ready for movement.

At the end of our LUNA YOGA session, relaxation allows the mind and body to integrate the experience fully. Stay in the final relaxation until your breath has become quiet and you are filled with a warm sense of comfort. Relaxing deeply at the end also helps release any residual tension and helps to avoid sore muscles. The effects of the exercises spread more deeply within and reverberate with more power when we relax completely afterward. If the exercises have stirred up memories or feelings, the final relaxation helps us come to a calm center.

It is vitally important to maintain the heat/energy/blood flow we have generated in the pelvic area for as long as possible at each LUNA YOGA session. If we immediately rush on to the next activity, the heat will flow away from the abdomen, and lessen the effectiveness of our practice. For instance, if we get up and walk around or run, the blood will flow into our legs; if we think, the energy will concentrate in the head; if we eat, the digestive organs will receive the heat. Thus it is crucial to relax fully, no matter how limited your time. Savor the sensations in your belly and slowly ease into your next activity after the relaxation. Or better yet, drink a cup of warm herbal tea after relaxing and before continuing with your day.

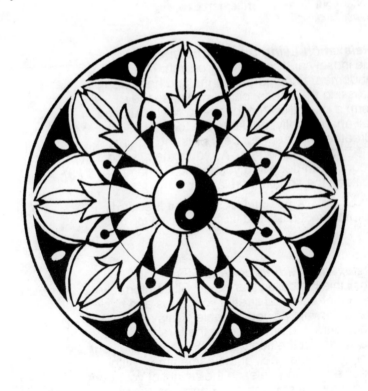

Relaxation Lying on the Back

Lie loosely and comfortably on your back on the floor. Let your legs fall open, a little more than shoulder width apart, toes pointing out. (This helps the back and pelvis relax.) Put your hands on your lower abdomen. Feel your breath there and bring your attention to this area. Let yourself sink completely in to Earth's gravity. Breathe deeply into your pelvis and belly.

Weed note: It's fine to put a pillow under your knees to further relax your lower back.

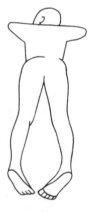

Relaxation Lying on the Abdomen

Lie loosely and comfortably on your abdomen, bringing your arms and hands up, crossing the hands, palms down, so they form a little pillow for your head. Let your legs fall apart slightly, but keep the toes touching. Breathe and feel your belly pressing against the floor as you inhale. As you exhale, send your breath deep into your back. Remember to keep the shoulders relaxed.

Weed note: A powerful energy circuit is created when the toes touch and the hands are on top of each other.

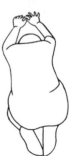

Relaxation Sitting on your Heels

I call this the coiled leaf pose. Sit comfortably on your heels and stretch your arms and back as far forward as you are able. Relax the shoulders and neck and let the forehead rest easily agaist the floor. Breathe deeply into your abdomen and back at the same time. With each exhalation, release the weight of your body ever more deeply into the Earth's embrace.

Variation on the Coiled Leaf

Again, sit on your heels, but this time spread your knees apart so your belly hangs loosely in between the thighs when you stretch the back and arms forward. Breathe deeply. Remember to focus on the belly and to keep the shoulders and neck relaxed.

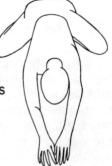

Weed note: If the shoulders are very tight, place a small pillow under the forehead only, keeping the arms on the floor.

Child's Pose Relaxation

The child's pose is similar to the coiled leaf, but the arms are relaxed towards the feet rather than stretched foward. Sit on your heels; keep your knees together or let them spread apart, as in the illustration, to leave more space for your belly (especially comfortable for pregnant women). Relax your arms along your sides and bend over until your forehead is on the floor. Keep the neck and shoulders totally relaxed. Breathe. This is an excellent position for those with a lot of tension in the back, and very calming for those dealing with upsetting emotions. (Also great for helping fidgety children relax.)

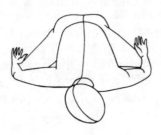

Breathing Techniques: Pranayama

Breathing techniques are called Pranayama, which means guidance of the breath. This does not mean we should constantly control and manipulate our breath. Breathing techniques rather serve to improve our perception of the flow of breath, allowing us to breathe more fully and naturally in every activity, not just LUNA YOGA.

Breathing keeps us alive, and creates a connection between the outer environment and the inner self. Breathing is the link between body, mind, and spirit.

In our culture a flat abdomen is seen as a sign of a fashionable figure. So we restrict our breathing to the chest, or in extreme cases, to the upper chest, so our bellies stay flat. But if we observe animals or babies, we see the belly moving and expanding with every breath. In our fear of obesity we restrict the breath and choke the energy which ought to circulate freely in the pelvis. It is extremely important in LUNA YOGA that you allow the belly to be raised and rounded when you inhale.

Pranayama offers many benefits. Simply to pay attention to our breathing can loosen up many muscle tensions, and even solve constipation. When we direct the breath deep into our pelvic area healing energy flows to the uterus, ovaries, bladder, and cervix. When we breathe deeply and regularly, we can stimulate the pituitary gland, which regulates our entire hormonal system.

Always remember to breathe through the nose. This retains and circulates the LUNA YOGA energy through the body. When we breathe through the open mouth, especially when it is done unmindfully, the energy is diverted from within and escapes to the outside. When we breathe through the nose, the air touches the inner skull and activates many parts of the brain.

In LUNA YOGA as in Hatha Yoga, the breath is always coordinated with our movements. When making an open movement, such as extended our arms or bending back or raising up, we inhale at the same time.

When we make a contracting or closing movement, like bending forward, we simultaneously exhale. The movements help the breath come and go like waves in the ocean, quietly, regularly, in our very own rhythm, regenerating us.

Although breathing is so simple that we do it every day, it is also very powerful. When done in conjunction with LUNA YOGA exercises, Pranayama can release old memories. Therefore, I advise you to find a person who is knowledgeable and experienced in Yoga, and ask them to guide you in your first experiences with Pranayama.

Here are the breathing exercises which I find most useful for LUNA YOGA.

Firebreath

This breathing technique stimulates (fires up) all metabolic processes. You can do it while standing, lying, sitting, squatting, or crouching on all fours. It has a very deep effect on the reproductive organs. Women who have an I.U.D. should not do this exercise—the I.U.D. could fall out!

Exhale completely, then pull the diaphragm up under the ribs. Remaining in full exhalation, push the diaphragm strongly down toward the pelvis. Without breathing, move the diaphragm up and down so your entire abdomen shakes in ripples. Possibly you can feel your uterus and other internal organs as they move. When you can't do this any longer, inhale again. Then take equal time to let your breath come and go in your own rhythm. The Firebreath can be repeated up to six times.

Subtle Breathing for the Third Eye

This form of breathing will invigorate both the pituitary and the pineal glands. Your entire body will feel sensitive and clear after this. Place index and middle finger of one hand on a point between your eyebrows, let your thumb and ring finger fall onto your nostrils and apply gentle pressure onto nose and forehead with your fingers. Let your breath flow in its own rhythm and observe your body sensations.

Weed note: Here are two Pranayama exercises I can share with you.

Alternate Nostril Breathing

This is a relaxing and centering breath, especially useful when you are stressed or emotionally upset.

Sit in a comfortable position with the spine straight. Curl the first and second fingers of the right hand in and tuck them into the fleshy part of the thumb's base as the thumb and ring and little fingers touch. Now bring this hand position up to your nose, with the thumb on the right side and the ring finger and little finger on the left side.

Gently press the right nostril closed with the thumb and inhale through the left nostril to a count of four. Now close the left nostril with gentle pressure from the fingers and retain the breath for a count of six. Release the thumb and exhale through the right nostril to a count of eight. Inhale through the right nostril to a count of four, then close it with the thumb and retain the breath for a count of six. Release the fingers and breathe out through the left nostril to a count of eight. This is one cycle.

Repeat the cycle as many times as you wish: inhale left for four; retain for six; exhale right for eight; inhale right for four; retain for six; exhale left for eight. As you become more at ease with alternate nostril breathing, you can lengthen the retention and exhalation, but keep the inhalation short. It doesn't matter which side you begin on, but always end the exercise on the same side on which you began.

Shakti Breath

This is an easier version of the firebreath, more suitable for beginners, but with the same benefits. Focus throughout on the diaphragm and abdomen. The Shakti breath is short and rapid, with all attention on the exhalation. The inhalation is allowed to happen without volition.

Sit in a comfortable position with the spine straight. Hands may be held loosely together in your lap, palms up; or in the mudra of univeral connection. To do the mudra (which means prayer with the hands), lay the forearms along the thighs with wrists over the knees, palms up. Lightly join the thumb and first finger in a circle and extend the other three fingers away from you.

Begin by inhaling deeply, expanding the belly fully. Then do one Shakti cycle: Exhale by pulling the diaphragm strongly up and forcing the air out of the nostrils in a gentle snort. Relax the diaphragm and allow the air to come in. A cycle will take one second or less. Do 20 cycles, ending with an exhalation. Do not breathe in; count to ten, then relax the diaphragm and inhale fully, letting the belly expand completely. Repeat up to three times.

As you become more proficient at the Shakti breath, you can increase the number of cycles you do. (30, 40 even 60!) You can also decrease the time per cycle, doing as many as two per second with an extremely forceful and rapid movement of the diaphragm. (It will sound like you are panting.) And, of course, you can lengthen the time of emptiness at the end, up to a full minute for the very advanced.

And the last word is Adelheid's:

Although there are many breathing techniques expounded in various books on Yoga, I consider Pranayama so precious and individual that I cannot in good conscience teach you any more than this via the written word. My fear is that you will slip into wrong habits unless you are personally guided. And incorrect breathing has very little healing quality. In my opinion, breathing exercises should be facilitated by an expert teacher who will make sure that you really know how to do them so healthy changes will develop and the breath will support you in becoming whole.

Gentle Sensing Exercises

The gentle sensing exercises are, in a manner of speaking, the daily bread (or muesli) of LUNA YOGA. I say this because these fairly easy and simple movements and positions can be done every day if desired.

The gentle sensing exercises bring us joy, give us energy, increase our vigor, and awaken our fertility and creativity.

These exercises are always synchronized with the rhythm of one's own breath. Please remember to be present with heart and soul.

As the name indicates, when doing these exercises we are sensing our own body and exploring the position and the condition of our inner organs, our muscles, our nerves, and our bones. The gentle sensing exercises facilitate a deep awareness of the interplay among body, mind, and spirit. As our awareness grows, we become more at ease with the many aspects of ourselves, and we can resonate more freely and easily with our desires and dislikes, our lust, our moods, with anything that may move us at the moment.

There are as many sensing exercises as there are human beings, because each individual will execute the exercises according to their own abilities. (Hatha Yoga, likewise, is said to include an infinite number of positions.) I have selected from the multitude of gentle sensing exercises those that are most useful for sensing the reproductive organs and the pelvis, the center of our vitality. They include exercises done while lying on the back, on the abdomen, in a sitting position, or crouching on all fours.

But you need not limit your practice to these exercises. As your pleasure in moving and sensing grows, you will automatically bring your imagination into play, and find yourself creating variations.

The body wants variety just like the mind and soul, not only in the daily menu, but also in posture and movement. All our senses want to be expressed and need material and spiritual nourishment. It feels good to try out different movements. Just as we eat every day and sleep every night and find our own rhythm in it, so does our body have desire for movement. Unfortunately, we often neglect it. We think about food because we are hungry and about sleep because we are tired. We have "unlearned" how to follow our natural instinct for movement—unlike children. It was driven out of us in the course of our socialization. Sit still in school, keep quiet in daily life, just don't be so conspicious!

It is good for us to build a regular time into our daily schedule for movement, and time for a conscious period of stillness. This allows our senses to unfold.

Gentle Sensing Exercises Lying on the Back

Crocodiles
These exercises strengthen the pelvic organs and increase the circulation of blood and energy into the uterus, ovaries, vagina, cervix, bladder, testes, and penis. The crocodile exercises also strengthen and comfort the spine, greatly easing lower back pain. They are ideal for those seeking to increase sexual responsiveness and pleasure.

A: Baby crocodile
Lie on your back; stretch your arms out to the sides. Sense your abdomen. Pull your knees up to your chest as you exhale. Continue exhaling as you roll the knees and hips to the right. (Knees will be close to your right elbow.) At the same time, turn your head to the left. Inhale and come back to center. Exhale and roll knees to the left, head to the right. Inhale as you return to center. This is a round. Do several rounds, always with the breath, until you feel loose and comfortable. Do one more round, remaining in each position for several breaths, feeling deeply into the pose.

(Translator's note: I have used "sense into it" or "feel into the pose" for German words that have no direct English translation. The German words illustrate the purpose of these exercises: to be still for a moment while holding a posture, and to "resonate" or "reverberate" witih the body sensation that has been created.)

B: Crocodile looks for food

Lie on your back, arms
extended to the sides. Bring
the knees up and put your feet on
the ground near your buttocks. Exhale
and roll your knees and hips to the right,
your head to the left. (It is ideal if the shoulders
remain flat on the floor.) Inhale, come to center.
Exhale, roll your knees and hips to the left, your
head to the right. Return to center. This is one
round. Do several rounds, always with the breath, until you feel
loose and comfortable. Then do one more round, remaining in
each position for several breaths, holding the pose and sensing
into it.

C. Crocodile swims slowly

Lie on your back, arms extended to the sides and
legs stretched slightly apart. Place the left foot
on the right knee. With your exhalation, roll
the left knee toward the floor on the right
and turn your head to look in the
opposite direction, toward your left hand.
(It is ideal if the shoulders stay in total
contact with the floor.) You may increase the
stretch by pressing the left knee to the floor with
your right hand. On your inhalation come to center
and with your exhalation bring the right foot on the left
knee and roll to the left. (Shoulders stay flat!) Inhale
and come center. This is one round. Do several rounds, always
with breath, until you feel loose and comfortable. Do one more
round, remaining in each position for several breaths, holding the
pose, sensing into it, and focusing your awareness on your belly.

D: *Crocodile swims quickly*

Lying on your back, arms outstretched, put the heel of the right foot on the toes of the left foot. Exhale and bring the right toes toward the floor on the left. Allow the movement to come from the hips, but keep the shoulders steady. At the same time, turn your head to the right. With your inhalation come back to center. Put the heel of the left foot on the toes of the right foot and bring the toes of the left foot toward the floor on the right as you exhale. Inhale as you return to center. This is one round. Practice several rounds. Remember to coordinate your movements with your breath. When you are relaxed and loose, do one more round, holding each position for a few breaths. Feel into it.

E: *Crocodile takes some sun*

Lie on your back legs extended, and stretch your arms to the sides. With your exhalation bring the left leg up and over the right leg until it reaches the right hand. Inhale and turn your head to the left. Breathe deeply into your pelvis and sense into it. Exhale and release to center. Inhale and relax. With the next exhalation, bring your right leg up and over your left leg until it reaches your left hand. Inhale and turn your head to the right. Breathe deeply and feel into your pelvis. Exhale and release to center.

F: *Crocodile shows off*

Lie on your back with legs extended and stretch your arms to the sides. With your exhalation bring your left leg up and out toward the left hand. With your inhalation release the leg and come to the center. Exhale and change sides. Practice the movement a few times, then hold the position for the length of a few breaths and sense into it.

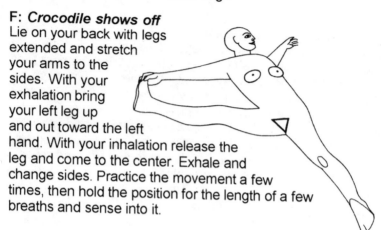

Pelvic Tilts and Tucks

Lying on your back, put your feet on the ground, so knees point upwards. With your exhalation, push your heels into the ground so your knees move slightly toward the toes, contract the muscles of your abdomen and pelvis and press your lower back strongly into the floor, so the pelvis tucks toward the chin. As you inhale, release the heels, relax the thighs and pelvic muscles, hollow your back slightly, push down on your buttocks and shoulders, and tilt your pelvis so your hip bones point toward your thighs. Do several tilts and tucks in the rhythm of your own breath. When you are easy with the positions, pause in each for a few breaths and sense how the pelvic organs shift as you tuck and tilt.

Bridge

Lying on your back, pull heels close to your buttocks. Hold the pressure points which increase blood and lymph circulation in the pelvis. (See page 119.) Allow knees to fall open. Tighten the muscles of the pelvic floor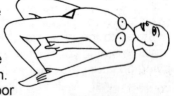
and lift the tailbone up slightly so the pelvis tilts toward the chin. As you exhale push against your shoulders and feet and raise your body up. Push out your belly button and try to touch it to the ceiling! Bring the elbows close together. As you exhale, roll down along your spinal column, from neck to tailbone. Practice this with a dynamic breath until you feel strong in it. Then hold each position for several breaths and allow yourself to feel deeply into your belly and spine. (Follow this with cuddle massage, p. 80.)

Chakrasana

This posture means "the wheel," which refers to our energy centers, known as wheels or chakras. It activates and harmonizes all the chakras of our body. Begin on your back, with legs extended and arms over your head. Bring your hands under your shoulders, fingers pointing toward toes, elbows up. Bring feet close to buttocks, knees pointing up. Lift your tailbone a little so your pelvis tilts toward the chin. Squeeze your anal sphincter and your vaginal muscles; contract entire pelvic floor and all the muscles there. Inhale and push strongly against your hands and feet, lifting your entire spine, even your head, off the floor. Make the belly as large and round as possible. Breathe deeply and feel. Exhale and gently lower yourself to the floor. Breathe and feel. Repeat once or twice if you wish. Follow with cuddle massage. Alternate: stand with your back to a wall, raise your arms, place your hands, fingers down, behind you; walk your hands down the wall to the floor, little by little, stepping away as you bend back. Breathe deeply and feel into it.

Cuddle Massage

This exercise relaxes your back and massages the sacral area (which is a reflex point for the entire pelvis). It is a "counter posture" to the bridge and the wheel and can be done anytime during your LUNA YOGA practice.

Lying on your back, pull your legs up to your chest. Make gentle circular movements with your lower back on the ground. First one direction, then the other. Don't forget to breathe!

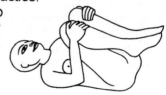

Slanted Ship

Lie on your back and fold your hands behind your neck. On your exhalation bring the right elbow and the left knee toward each other. The left elbow stays on the floor, as does the right leg, which is fully extended, ankle flexed. With your inhalation come back to the beginning position. Exhale and bring the left elbow and right knee toward each other, keeping the right elbow and left leg firmly on the floor. Practice this movement a few times; then hold each side for several breaths while you feel into it.

Lying Split

Lie on your back with legs fully extended. Relax on your inhalation and raise the left leg. As you exhale, grasp the thigh, or knee, or ankle, and pull the leg toward you. Lift your head and draw the knee toward the nose. Keep the right leg firmly down, outstretched on the ground, with foot flexed. Breathe deeply and sense fully for a breath or two. Release the leg as you exhale. Repeat with right leg.

Gentle Sensing Exercises in Sitting Positions

Sensing exercises in sitting position are more strenuous than those done lying down, but generate more energy in the pelvis. While the sitting exercises work the entire body, they are especially effective at restoring and nourishing strong flows of nervous system energy into the reproductive organs, and help us focus intently on the abdomen. Be sure to use your attention and breath to direct the energy deep into your abdomen and pelvis as you do these exercises. Because many of them stretch and twist the spine, I advise you to relax for a few breaths after every exercise, allowing any tension in your back to loosen up and the energy you have generated to flow down into the belly.

Butterfly

This is a series of exercises with many variations, for the Butterfly, symbol of metamorphosis, knows all kinds of tricks.

A: *Butterfly spreads its wings*

Sit up with your spine erect and shoulders relaxed. Pull your feet in toward your trunk, soles together. Knees fall outward toward the floor. Breathe and sense into your pelvis. Hands are placed on the knees, and, with a little gentle pressure, you can assist and extend this powerful opening stretch.

B: *Butterfly looks over a flower*
While sitting in the Butterfly position, place
the right hand on the left knee. Reach
your left hand and arm as far back
toward the right buttock as you can,
placing it on the floor behind you,
fingers down. Allow the entire upper
body to twist so you look back over
your left shoulder. Hold for a few
breaths, feeling into your spine and
belly. Repeat on the opposite side.

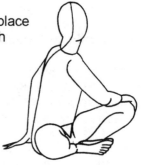

C: *Butterfly finds a flower;*
** *it is far away***
   While sitting in the Butterfly position,
slide the feet forward about a foot.
Stretch your arms and trunk forward and
down.   Stretch out of your lower back
and hips—with forearms in front of your
shins—and sense the energy moving in
your pelvis as the sacrum opens.

D: *Butterfly finds a flower close by*
Begin with the Butterfly, the soles of the feet
touching. Pull heels as close to the
genitals as possible. Stretch forward
and down to sip nectar from the
flower. Let each exhalation carry
you a bit further into the stretch. Don't
rock. Breathe into the belly.

E: *Butterfly becomes frolicsome*

Start out in the Butterfly position, but this time hold your feet with your hands. As you exhale, roll backwards along your spine; as you inhale, come back into position. Try it at different speeds, but always with the breath. Feel how the pelvis responds to the rocking of the different rhythms. Sense in to your body.

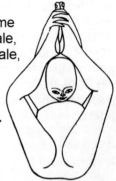

F: *Butterfly rests and pulses its wings*

Assume the Butterfly pose, holding the feet with the hands. Roll onto your back. Exhale and turn your head to the right, letting your left knee and pelvis roll to the left side. Inhale and come back to center. With the next exhalation, turn your head to the left and let your right knee and pelvis roll to the right side. Try different speeds, maintaining the connection to your breath. Sense the organs of the pelvis. How do they respond to this?

G: *Butterfly sleeps and has a dream*

Hold the feet in the Butterfly pose and roll onto your back. With your exhalation pull up your head, with your inhalation put it back down. Keep the shoulders and neck relaxed. Practice dynamically for a few times, then hold the position for several breaths and feel into the pose.

H: *Butterfly touches the earth*

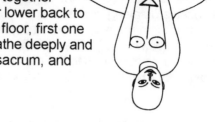

Lie on your back in the Butterfly position, holding the feet together with the hands. Use your lower back to draw small circles on the floor, first one way, then the other. Breathe deeply and sense into the tailbone, sacrum, and genitals.

J: *Butterfly takes a sunbath*

Roll onto your back with legs and feet in Butterfly position. Best if thighs remain in contact with the floor. Breathe out and use your hands to press your thighs gently down and outward. Inhale and relax the pressure. After a few flutters up and down, remain in the fully stretched position for several breaths and feel into the exposed belly.

K: *Butterfly does yoga*

Roll onto your back in Butterfly pose and bring your hands behind your neck, interlacing your fingers. Exhale and bring the left elbow and right knee together. Inhale and relax; lie back down. Exhale and bring the right elbow and left knee together. Inhale and relax. Move rhythmically for several breaths, then hold each position for a few breaths and feel into your body.

L: *Butterfly does a mating dance*
Remain lying down in the Butterfly pose,
hands folded behind your head. Relax
head and neck completely. Pick up
head up with hands as you exhale.
(DO NOT USE YOUR NECK to lift
your head.)   Inhale and lower your hands, thus lowering the
head, back to the floor. Practice several times dynamically, then
keep the head held up (relax that neck!) and feel into the pose,
while breathing deeply.

M: *Butterfly looks for a mate*
Lie on your back in Butterfly pose,
with hands behind your neck. As
you inhale, use your hands to
lift your head and turn it to the
right. Breathe deeply, and feel
into this. Then use your hands
to turn your head to the left side.
Again, breathe deeply and feel into it.

N: *Butterfly finds a mate and
is very happy*
Remain in Butterfly pose on your back
with your fingers interlaced behind the
neck. As you exhale, bring elbows
and knees together. As you inhale,
return to the lying pose. Keep the
neck very relaxed. Practice dynamically, moving with the breath, for a while.
Then hold the pose, breathing deeply and sensing into your
body.

*After all these Butterflies, stretch out on your back and relax
deeply for a full minute or more, sensing any changes in your
reproductive organs.*

Sitting Triangles: Trikonasana

Triangles help us become more grounded, down to earth, and stable. Most triangles are done standing; these two variations are best done sitting. A triangle pointing down is an ancient symbol for female (specifically for female genitals, the yoni). Note how Esther Lisette Ganz, the illustrator, has used the triangle in her figures. (And note that she uses the ancient symbol for the sun, still used by today's astrologers, to indicate the breasts.) When doing these exercises, envision the triangles you are making, and focus on your own yoni and pelvic area.

A: *Triangle twist*

Sit on your feet, with knees spread wide apart. Place the right hand on the left knee; stretch the left arm and hand around and back toward the right buttock, letting your head follow the arm and shoulder so you wind up looking backwards over your shoulder. Breathe deeply and feel into the pose. Repeat with left hand on right knee, stretching the right arm toward the left buttock. Breathe and feel into your belly.

B: *Triangle stretch*

Sit on your feet, with knees apart, inhale, raise your arms and interlace your fingers behind your neck. As you exhale, slowly lower your right elbow toward your right knee and bend to the side, keeping your back straight. Breathe deeply. Inhale and return to upright and center. Exhale and slowly lower your left elbow toward your left knee. Practice several times dynamically, then hold each side for a few deep and long breaths while experiencing the power of the triangle.

Rocking the baby

Sit straight up, with legs loosely crossed. Flex and bring in your left leg, so the heel is as close as possible to the vulva.   Take your right leg in your arms: your foot rests in your left elbow and your knee in the right elbow. Rock your leg like a baby, breathe deeply, and feel into your body, your pelvis, your yoni. Repeat with the right heel tucked in the vulva and the left leg held and rocked while you breathe and sense. Continue with "Toe to Nose."

Toe to nose greeting

After doing one or more rounds of "Rocking the Baby," lift each leg in turn and bring the big toe of the foot you are cradling right up to your nose. Do not bend your neck. Do not bring your nose toward your toe. Keep your back straight. Breathe for several deep breaths and sense into your hips and belly.   Continue with "Foot to Head."

Foot to head greeting

After completing "Toe to Nose" on both sides, sit up very straight and stretch your legs straight out. Flex the left knee and place the left heel close into the crotch. Guide your right leg up (the leg is outside the arms) and with your hands place the foot over your head. Breathe and feel deeply into this posture, into your inner pelvic stuctures.

Arrows

The arrow exercises give a deep stretch to the backs of the legs and the inner thighs. This strengthens the veins and helps prevent varicose veins. Arrow stretches also open the pelvic area and increase the amount of energy flowing into the womb.

A: *Straight arrow*

Sit straight up with legs extended in front of you. Bring your left foot in, close to your vulva. Breathe out, grasp your right leg with both hands and draw it straight up, knee to nose. Keep your back straight. Inhale and release. Repeat several times with the right leg, then hold while you breathe deeply and sense into your belly for 1-3 breaths. Change legs and repeat the entire sequence.

B: *Broken arrow*

Sit straight up, legs extended in front of you. Breathe in and bring the left foot toward the body; hold the ankle with the right hand. Breathe out, grasp the right leg with the left hand and gently, but firmly, stretch it toward the left. Inhale back to center. Do this several times in tune with your own breathing, then hold for 1-3 breaths and experience the sensations in your belly and body. Repeat by holding right ankle in left hand and stretching left leg to the right with the right hand.

C: *Wide arrow*

Sit straight up; legs extended in front of you. Flex your left knee and bring your left foot close to the genitals; hold your knee with your left hand. Stretch the right leg to the right side and, while consciously breathing, grasp your right toes with your right hand. Gently, but firmly, stretch your leg up and further toward the right. Breathe fully and release. Repeat several times before holding the pose and sensing into it. Then, bring the right knee in and stretch the left leg out. Repeat.

(Note: I can't tell you exactly when to inhale and exhale in this exercise because your breathing will change with planetary and lunar influences.)

Crab

The crab position increases blood circulation in the pelvic organs, and stretches the back. It is a soothing position which strongly supports our efforts to increase awareness of the pelvic/genital area. Sit up quite straight and bring your feet together in front of you, heels into genitals. Reach underneath your flexed legs and grasp your calves, or ankles, or feet. Lean over and rest the head and neck on the feet or floor. Breathe deeply for ten breaths. Sense fully, noting where you feel tension, what you are hearing in your mind, how easy (or not) it feels to have your face close to your genitals, close enough to look at them, close enough to smell them.

Tortoise

Sit with legs spread about
eighteen inches apart, knees
slightly flexed. Exhale as you
bend forward and down,
extending your shoulders and
arms. Inhale in this position. Exhale
and reach your hands underneath your
legs back to your buttocks, palms up. Extend head and feet
forward. Relax your head, your neck, your upper back, and
your lower back. Let your chin or forehead rest on the floor.
Breathe and feel into your pelvis. Be as slow as a tortoise.

Pachimottasana

Pachimottasana exercises are ones in which the back is well
stretched (the literal translation of the Sanskrit word means
"extending the back"). Traditionally these exercises are
recommended for those whose energy is erratic, or lacking in
vitality. Pachimottasana exercises also have a reputation for
increasing the beauty and grace of the body, as well as helping
to rejuvenate sexuality.

A: Full forward bend

Sit straight and upright. Stretch your back up, stretching strongly
out of the lower back (the lumbo-sacral area). Expand the spine
as you inhale. Exhale; stretch your legs forward, keeping your
knees as straight as possible. Inhale and lift your arms over your
head. Exhale and bend forward and
down. Move slowly and with
awareness and breathe deeply
into the pose. If it is too much of a
strain to keep your legs straight,
you may bend the knees.

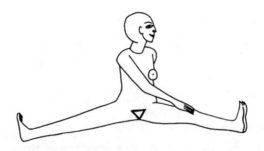

B: *Split twist*

Sit straight and open the spine while you inhale. Exhale. Then spread your legs wide as you inhale. Lay your right hand on your left knee, bring your left hand backwards to the right buttock, looking back over the left shoulder. Breathe deeply and sense your spine and your belly in this twist. Exhale and relax. Repeat with left hand on right knee, right hand to left buttock, looking over your right shoulder.

C: *Sideways forward bend*

Sit up straight. Raise your arms and hands over your head as you inhale and open your legs into a very wide **V**. Turn your entire upper body to the right. Exhale; stretch your trunk and arms forward and down, chin toward knee, elbows toward floor. Breathe and sense deeply into your body in this position. Inhale and return to upright. Turn to the left and repeat.

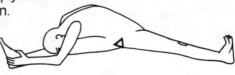

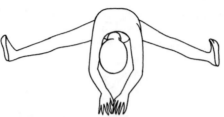

D: *Split forward bend*

Sit with your legs in a split; breathe in and lift your arms overhead. As you exhale, bend forward and down. Stop and inhale, no matter how little you've moved, before exhaling and continuing to stretch forward and down. If you can't reach the floor, it's fine to use a large firm cushion for some support. If you can reach the floor, pull yourself forward with your arms to increase the stretch. Relax slightly into a comfortable expansion forward. Breathe fully into the pelvis and spine and sense fully into yourself.

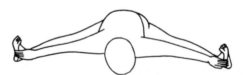

E: *Eagle forward bend*

Sit with your legs spread apart. Exhale and reach with your hands toward each foot. Inhale, then use your arms to pull yourself further down and forward with each exhalation. After three or four breaths, relax slightly into a comfortable expansion, breathe deeply and sense into your spine and pelvic area for several breaths.

F: *Spiral half-twist*

Sit up very straight. Pick up the right foot and lay it on the left thigh, sole up. (On the floor is fine if you can't reach the thigh or can't comfortably keep your foot there.)

Reach the right hand behind your back to grab your right foot, or your left thigh if your foot is on the floor. Place the left hand on the right knee. Look far back over your right shoulder. Breathe and sense deeply into yourself. Repeat with your left foot on right thigh, left arm behind to grasp your left foot (or right thigh), right hand on left knee, looking over your left shoulder, breathing.

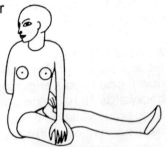

G: *Half-lotus forward bend*

Sit up very straight; breathe deeply. Pick up the right foot and lay it on the left thigh. Inhale and bring both arms overhead. Exhale and fold forward from the hips with the foot still resting on the thigh. Stretch your hands forward to the foot of your straight leg, grasp your toes, or ankle, and pull yourself forward with each inhalation, stretching forward out of your lower back. After several breaths, relax slightly into a comfortable extension. Breathe deeply and feel your pelvis, your belly.

Backward Bends

After we do Pachimottasana/forward bends, it is important give the spine the opposite impulse. Thus, here are postures of backward bending. (See also *Bridge* pose and *Wheel* pose, both on page 79.)

Slanted Plane
Sit up very straight and place your hands, palms down, next to you, fingertips pointing backwards. Inhale and push your body up so you are balanced on hands and heels. Breathe deeply, sensing into your body.

Camel
Kneel and come to your center. Breathe in, expand the chest and shoulders, and begin to arc backwards slightly. Rest at each exhale; and with each inhale bend further back, stretching your hands toward your heels. Let your breath stream into your pelvis.

Cow

The asanas I call Cows strengthen the entire pelvic area and help nourish excellent functioning of the pelvic/sexual organs. Like the Butterfly and Crocodile, there are many variations of the Cow. Here are a few of my favorites.

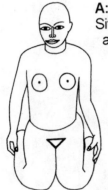

A: *Contented Cow*
Sit between your legs with a straight spine and rock or sway from side to side. This has a beneficial effect on the legs as well as the pelvis.

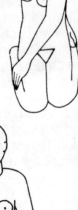

B: *Adventuresome Cow*
Sit between your legs, exhale, and reach the right hand back to the left foot, placing the left hand on the right knee. Look over your right shoulder. Sense into this as you breathe deeply. After a few breaths change sides.

C: *The Cow's Horns*
Cross your legs, left thigh on top, bringing your knees over each other so the calves extend out the sides. Grasp your feet or ankles in your hands. Sway from side to side and breathe deeply. How do you feel? How does your pelvis feel? Recross legs so the right thigh is on top and repeat.

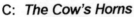

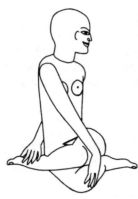

D: *Cow in a tight place*

Begin in Cow's horns, left thigh on top. Exhale and turn to the left, bringing the left hand behind the back to catch the left toes/foot. Support yourself with your right hand on your right knee, and look back over your left shoulder. Breathe deeply and feel into this position. Repeat on the other side.

E: *Classic Cow*

Cross your legs to make the Cow's Horns, left thigh on top. Pull your feet in as close to your sides as possible. Perhaps you can even sit on both feet.   Reach the right arm high overhead as you inhale. Bend your right elbow and grasp the left hand which reaches to it from behind the back. Exhale. Stretch and breathe deeply. Feel into yourself. Relax the arms. Raise the left arm with your inhale. Reach the right one up to it and let them join behind the back. Breathe and sense. Recross your legs, so the right thigh is on top.   Repeat both arm positions, so you practice a total of four variations.

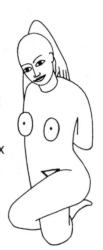

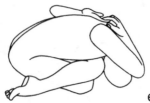

F: *Cow grazes*

Begin with any of the four positions of the Classic Cow. Bend forward and down. Breathe and sense deeply into your pelvic genital area. Repeat in each different arm and leg position.

Squat

This is a classical position from Hatha Yoga. It releases the back, strengthens the pelvic floor, and aids digestion. It is a powerful ally in focusing your attention on your abdomen and reproductive organs. This is a very important exercise for those who wish to increase fertility or sexual pleasure. Begin by standing up very straight, feet parallel and about hip-width apart. With the heels on the

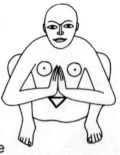

floor, bend your knees and lower your rear toward the floor, breathing out and keeping the back as straight as possible. Push your knees apart with your elbows, or wedge your upper body in between your knees, bringing your elbows in front of your calves and placing your palms together. Breathe. Sense deeply into the genitals and pelvis.

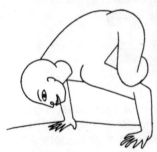

Crow

When you can do the Squat with ease, try this. Begin in a squat. Place your hands on the floor in front of you, fingers spread and pointing forward, with elbows sharply bent. Lean forward until the knees come to rest on your arms and you are balanced on your hands. Hold the balance with deep and regular breathing.

Pheasant

After the Squat and the Crow, you can try this. Place your hands strongly in front of you, fingers wide and pointed forward. Breathe in and push yourself up with your arms, swinging your legs to the left and balancing them on your left arm. Breathe out, relax in the position and sense deeply.

Gentle Sensing Exercises Lying Face Down

Doing exercises lying on the stomach works the back quite strongly. The pressure helps strengthen digestive and reproductive functions, as well as directing our attention into the belly.

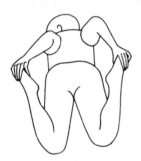

Flat Boat
Lie on your abdomen, flex your knees, inhale, and reach your hands back to grab your feet. On exhalation, press your feet out from your buttocks toward the floor. Repeat several times. Then relax and breathe deeply.

Cobra
Lie on your belly, place your hands under your shoulders, fingers pointing forward, with elbows bent up. Inhale and smoothly roll up, starting with the eyes; then lift forehead, chin, shoulders, and finally, the upper body. Do not lock or straighten your elbows. Relax the shoulders. Stretch and bend backward. Breathe deeply and sense into your belly.

When you are comfortable with this pose, increase the difficulty by beginning with your hands clasped under your forehead, instead of under your shoulders, as in the illustration. Push up, hold, and breathe deeply.

All Cobra poses are beneficial to the inner organs.

Swan

Lie on your belly, place your hands under your shoulders, with elbows bent up, and flex your knees, feet pointing upwards. Inhale and smoothly roll up: roll your eyes up, lift your forehead, lift your chin, lift your upper body. Do *not* lock or straighten your elbows. Relax your shoulders. Breathe deeply, sense into your body, and afterwards relax well.

Locust

Lie on your abdomen, inhale and lift your right leg up, supporting it at the knee with the left foot. Breathe deeply and sense into your pelvis. Exhale, release. Inhale and lift your left leg, supporting it at the knee with the right foot. Breathe deeply and sense into your pelvis. Exhale, release.

Rocking Boat

Lie on your abdomen, inhale and reach your hands back to grab your feet. Exhale. On the next inhalation, pull the arms and legs away from each other and raise the thighs and upper body into the air. Stay in this full extension and breathe, noting how the breath rocks your body like a little boat on the sea. This exercise strengthens abdominal muscles, improves functioning of kidneys and bladder, and, of course, strongly benefits the sexual organs. (To release shins, flex toes away from head.)

Gentle Sensing Exercises on All Fours

Exercises on all fours are some of the best for deepening your awareness of your pelvic region. These sensing exercises are gentle and strong at the same time.

Cat

Cats are associated with the moon. These exercises help us connect with the sensuous energy of the cat.

Weed note: The cat, who always seems to move with grace, focused intention, and powerful body awareness is a wonderful archetypal ally to help us reclaim and remember our bodies and our bellies.

A: *Simple Cat*
(No illustration.)
Kneel on hands and knees, with hands directly under shoulders, and knees directly under hips. Breathe in and lift the head and chest up, expanding and opening the chest as much as possible. (Let your back sway down like an old horse). Breathe out and let your head go down toward the floor, between the arms, while the back arches up like a frightened or angry cat. Repeat, following the breath, several times. If you like, try it faster and try it very slowly. Breathe and sense fully into the sacrum and the pelvis.

B: *Happy Cat*
Kneel on all fours, aligned as in the Simple Cat. With your inhalation, lift your left leg, turn to the left, and look backwards. Exhale and release. Inhale and repeat three times before switching sides and lifting the right leg, looking back and to the right.

C: *Playful Cat*

Kneel on all fours, aligned as in the Simple Cat. With your exhalation bring your right knee up to your right elbow, and bend your head down to your right elbow. Breathe deeply and sense into your pelvis. Repeat, bringing your left knee up to your left elbow, and your head down to that elbow.

Deep Forward Stretch

Kneel on all fours. Breathe out and reach forward with your hands, stretching until the buttocks are well raised. Keep the hips and knees in a line. With each exhalation, bring the chest a little nearer to the floor. Breathe deeply and enjoy the pose as you sense fully into your genitals/pelvis.

Dog

Kneel on all fours, with the hands placed so the thumbs point forward, the fingers point out to the side, shoulder width apart. Inhale and push up with the arms and legs. Breathe deeply into the back and allow it to lengthen without sagging. Push the heels to the floor as you exhale. Relax the shoulders, but do not let the head hang. Breathe deeply and sense into the pelvis. Hold the position as long as it feels comfortable.

Moon

This exercise represents the moon in all of her phases. As opposed to the previous exercises, which are done as separate positions, this one is done as one complete, smooth, flowing action. It deepens our emotional life, and helps us to deal with moods and sentiments. It has a deep nourishing effect on the pelvic organs and refines our appearance as well.

Crescent moon

Kneel on hands and knees with hands under shoulders and knees under hips and bring the right foot up between your hands. Stretch the left leg far back. Energy is centered and focused in the pelvis, the balance point between the hands and the extended foot.

Waxing moon

Place your hands on your right knee. Breathe deeply for several breaths and feel the energy focused in your pelvis.

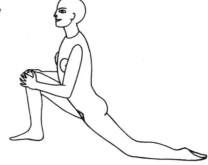

Full moon

Keeping your attention and your energy focused deep in your pelvis, inhale, raise your arms and bend back. Breathe deeply into your abdomen/pelvis. Continue for several breaths.

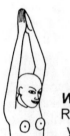

Waning moon

Release your arms to the ground as you sit down on your left foot, with the right leg extended. Stretch your arms upward and breathe deeply for several breaths.

New moon

Bend forward over the right leg as you exhale, grasping the toes with your hands and bringing your chin to your knee. Breathe deeply, stretch softly, and sense fully into the pelvis/genitals. Release.

Repeat the entire sequence (all five moon phases) beginning with Crescent moon with the left leg between your hands.

Pelvic Floor Exercises (Kegels)

Although they are not specifically part of LUNA YOGA, I believe (and so do all the professionals who reviewed this manuscript), that pelvic floor exercises are a vital component of any program that seeks to establish reproductive health and sexual well-being. Classical yoga includes one such exercise, the "anal sphincter lock" or *Moola Bandha*.

Pelvic floor exercises—commonly known after Doctor Kegel, who made them an important part of his practice in helping women with reproductive (and urinary) problems—are focused on tonifying the deep internal muscles of the pelvis. They can be done while you are doing the gentle sensing exercises (during the passive sensing breaths), as a separate part of your LUNA YOGA practice, or at odd times of the day.

First locate and feel your pelvic floor (PF) muscles, including: the muscles around the anus, the muscles of the vagina, the muscles around the neck of the urinary bladder, and the muscles supporting the uterus and intestines. If you are uncertain of where these are, here's one way to feel them: stop your stream of urine when you're voiding. Another way is to place your finger into the vagina and tighten your muscles around it. Once you've located the muscles, exercise them.

Basic Tonifying Kegel: Breathe in and tighten the PF muscles. Hold and sense for 3-13 seconds. Then breathe out and release. This is one pulse. A round is ten pulses. Ten rounds a day is recommended.

Butterfly Kegel: Pulse the PF muscles rapidly, tightening and releasing them at least once every second, faster if you can. Continue for at least one minute.

Water Kegel: Sit in a basin or bathtub with water up to your hips. See if you can draw water into your vagina as you breathe in; forcefully expel the water as you exhale. Continue for at least a minute.

This entire page is a Weed note.

Some Notes on Hatha Yoga

I started to study Yoga as a student in Vienna in 1967. Different teachers that I studied with emphasized different aspects in their courses: sometimes my Yoga classes had a strictly spiritual focus, at other times they were related solely to the body; some teachers had a playful approach, others were strict; one stressed discipline, while another valued creativity.

In 1978 I started training as a Yoga teacher. This laid the basis for further education in different body therapies. The female body—my own!—became the focus of my attention when, in the early eighties, I was diagnosed with cervical cancer. How could this happen to me? I'd lived a healthy lifestyle for so long! Shock, disillusionment, reflection and pondering took turns.

I had a vague idea that being fully alive was expressed in changing moods and had nothing in common with mechanical monotony. I turned my attention away from my job and toward my cycle.

I looked closely at my fears that had to do with being a woman, and I began to wonder what I would really enjoy doing. I wanted to live with lust and as I pleased, and not fight and compete. I did not want to prove anything, just live and be. I pursued the path of Yoga.

Through dealing with my ill-being I arrived at my well-being. And my specific disease also showed me a special way to my womanhood, a new/old Yoga I call LUNA YOGA.

In many classical schools of Yoga there are strict rules; there are few rules in LUNA YOGA.

In classical Yoga in eastern India it is still common to place strict discipline on the student. Aviva Steiner arranged her menstrual calisthenics according to strict rules. But our western world of work produces so many rules that I felt something curative could grow better for me out of open chaos.

Visiting the United States, I found women freely adapting old traditions. I experienced ancient revered arts which were viewed with curiosity rather than complete acceptance, and ideas which were tested for their suitability, no matter how ancient. What felt good, what nourished beauty was accepted; whatever was not beneficial was left out. In this way, I saw old traditions come to life again and give good results for contemporary people.

Without strict rules, the varied gender roles for women and men in different countries and cultures, now as well as in herstory, open up new outlooks for the shaping of our own lives, allowing women, especially, more freedom of expression, more ways to be recognized as fertile and creative.

LUNA YOGA borrows freely from Hatha Yoga, and encourages you to try out and to acquire new forms of movement. Many ideas streaming in indirectly, as well as directly through my teachers, have nourished LUNA YOGA from within. Its structure has shaped itself, its forms have stabilized and liquefied again.

The movement arts in old traditions often exhibit some similarities. Is this an expression that the human body has remained unchanged in the course of millennia? Many schools of movement emphasize right measure and moderation; they point out again and again the interchange between tension and relaxation, cycles and rhythms, fixed forms as well as spontaneous, impulsive activities. All are opportunities to arrive at well-being, are they not? May your journey with these exercises be one of wholeness.

Fertility Dances

The fertility dance exercises are the feast of LUNA YOGA. Just as you wouldn't give a banquet every day, you don't do fertility dances on a daily basis. Too much of a powerful thing does not lead to good health. In the traditions of the tribal people who originated these (modified) dances, fertility dances and fertility rituals are allowed only at specific, defined times.

These vigorous fertility dances stimulate ovulation, deepen sexual sensation, can bring on menstruation, and improve sperm count and quality. In combination with the Gentle Sensing Exercises they are highly effective when performed as directed.

Any attempt to do these dances will benefit you, but for greatest benefit, look for a teacher who can get you off to a good start. Whether you have a teacher or not, be sure to limit your practice to the times I specify and to the ways I suggest the dances be done. You can, of course choose your own sequence of steps and thus make up your own unique fertility dance.

The fertility dance exercises need to be done with attention to detail. Every motion has meaning: the movements of the arms convey messages, the bending of the head evokes feelings, and the rocking of the pelvis generates and circulates Shakti, the great force of all life.

In the African people I found a delight in movement. I admired their lusty willingness to frisk and caper and to surrender to the impulses of their bodies. And I especially noted their ability to stay in one's own rhythm. Perhaps they took it in with their mother's milk, but it can be learned. We can learn it. We can learn to move freely. We can learn not just about staying with oneself, in one's own center, but also about entering into encounter, about moving in contact and communication with others. We can move with passion and delight, not just to dance on feast days and celebrations, but in our daily lives as well.

When we dance, we must breathe with attention, inhaling and exhaling through the nose. This helps us coordinate the movements of our bodies with the unique rhythm of our breath. Inhale as you open, exhale when you close.

The movements of the fertility dances don't have to be done quickly. If your breathing rhythm is slow, move slowly. However, it is important to keep the movement flowing and uninterrupted, so it can send a strong impulse to the physiological processes of the body, especially to the hormonal system.

Note: If your intention is to hinder implantation of a fertilized egg, you have to execute the dances as soon as possible after fertilization has occurred and at precise 24-hour intervals for the next four days, with forceful exhalation through the nose, and with stamping feet. (See page 127 for full sequence.)

If your intention is to increase fertility, step more lightly, and do the dances only before ovulation has occurred. (See page 125 for full sequence.)

Basic Fertility Dance Steps

Basic Fertility Dance Stance
(No illustration)
Place your feet parallel (neither turned inward nor outward) about hip distance apart. Keep your pelvis relaxed, and your knees slightly flexed (not locked or rigid). Let the shoulders and arms also relax. Maybe it will help you to imagine a chair behind you: assume a posture as if you were about to sit down. Let your breath sink deeply into your abdomen and pelvis. Sense into the stance.

Pelvic Turns
Begin in the basic fertility dance stance, described above. Inhale and bring the hands to rest on the hips. Exhale and turn to the right. Inhale to center. Exhale and turn to the left. Sense into the pelvis. Initiate these turns from your sacroiliac joint, but extend them all the way to the top of the head. Your sacroiliac joint is between your hipbones and your sacrum. You can best feel this little joint when you place your hand on your sacrum and feel with your fingers for the indentations in this flattened bone. Turn left and right and see if you can feel the movement in the joint.

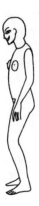

Weight Shifting #1
Assume the basic fertility dance stance, arms relaxed. Breathe fully into the pelvis, letting the abdomen round out. As you breathe, shift your weight from center to back and back to center and to the front and back to the basic dance stance. Keep your center of gravity deep in the pelvis. Breathe and sense thoroughly into your womb.

Weight Shifting #2

Assume the basic fertility dance stance and breathe completely into the pelvis. Shift your weight as far to the right as you can. Return to center. Shift as far to the left as you can. Return to center. Continue, keeping your breath flowing out of a soft, open pelvis.

Weight Shifting #3

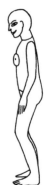

Begin in the basic fertility dance stance. Breathing fully, shift your weight to the left, then to the front. Inhale and continue shifting your weight to the right, and then to the back so you've drawn an imaginary small circle in the air (parallel to the floor) with your pubic bone. Do this as one continuous motion, inhaling and exhaling as you shift the weight of your pelvis in a circle to the right. After several repetitions, shift to the left. Sense totally into the pelvis/genitals.

Belly Dances

Belly dance is an ancient oriental tradition of dances which prepared women for healthy pregnancies and safe births by strengthening and opening their pelvic structures (muscles, ligaments, bones).

Traditionally, belly dances were done only by women for women, but today we can all do belly dances, for both women and men want to strengthen their pelvic structures and deepen their sexual sensations and pleasures.

Here are a few basic forms to begin with. If you intend to use these exercises to bring on your menstruation, then you must thrust your pelvis very forcefully and exhale with much passion. If your goal is to stimulate fertility, your movements have to be more gentle.

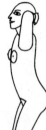

Beginning Belly

Begin by assuming the basic fertility dance stance. You may cross your hands behind your neck, or extend your arms to the sides, or place your hands on your hips. Inhale, keep the back and shoulders still and tilt your pelvis back by pointing your pubic bone toward the floor.

Exhale and rock your pelvis forward by tilting your pubic bone up toward the ceiling.

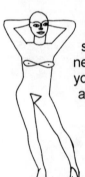

Next Belly

Assume the basic fertility dance stance, with your hands behind your neck, out to the sides, or on your hips. Breathe into your pelvis and sense deeply and fully. Keep your attention there as you breathe out, relax your left knee, push with your right foot, and rock your pelvis to the left. Inhale back to center. Breathe out, relax the right knee, push slightly with the left foot, and shift your pelvis to the right. Feet do not move.

Full Belly Roll

Take the basic fertility dance stance, with your arms behind neck, on hips (akimbo), or relaxed at your sides. Inhale and focus fully into the pelvis/hips. Move smoothly to the right, making a small circle with your pubic bone while inhaling. As you exhale, make a forceful pelvic thrust. Inhale and move smoothly to the left, making a small circle with your pubic bone. Exhale with a forceful forward pelvic thrust.

Windmill

Assume the basic fertility dance stance. Inhale and raise your right arm up, tilt your buttocks backward (point pubic bone toward floor), bend your head back, and stretch the left arm down.

With your exhalation let your head fall forward, tuck your pelvis forward (pubic bone toward the ceiling), switch arms, so the left arm is stretched up and the right arm is stretched down.

Feel the stretch coming from the pelvic floor. Let your attention be finely focused on the abdomen. Try various speeds, always coordinating with your own breathing. Go at a pace you can sustain for many minutes. Yes, slow is fine.

Circus Jump

Stand in the basic fertility dance stance, with relaxed arms. When you inhale, jump out of the basic stance and turn at least half way around with your knees remaining flexed. With your exhalation, come back to the ground—forcefully if you want to bring on menstruation; gently if you want to stimulate fertility. Repeat several times on each side.

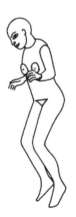

Monkey Business

From the basic fertility dance stance, exhale
and bend down, letting your trunk rest on
your thighs. Head and arms dangle easily
onto the floor, palms up. Keep the knees
soft and relaxed and at least partly bent.
When you inhale, lift your right leg as if to
take a step; the knee pushes up on the passive
chest, the arm dangles. Exhale and step
down: softly for fertility, with a stomp for initiat-
ing menstruation. Inhale and raise the left leg,
pushing the chest up. Exhale as the foot
returns to the floor.

Monkey and Banana

From the basic fertility dance
stance, exhale and bend down,
resting your torso on your thighs.
Do not let the head dangle in this posture: keep the neck extended and in line
with the rest of the spine. Stretch one arm to
the front, the other arm back. Keep the knees
easily bent. When you inhale, take a step forward with one
foot, extend one arm and bring the other arm back. When you
exhale, extend one arm, bring the other arm back and step
back. You can do this exercise all different ways: left arm, left
foot; right arm, right foot; left arm, right foot; and right arm, left
foot. If you want to bring on menstruation, your step has to be
forceful and stomping. Step lightly for support of your fertility.

Harvest Dance

Begin in the basic fertility dance stance. With your inhalation, open your arms far to the sides and open your fingers wide, extend your head back, tilt your buttocks back (pubic bone looks down), and step one leg (alternate left and right) to the side, with your knee bent and your foot straight.

On your exhalation, let your head fall forward, bring your hands together, make fists and bring them to your pelvis. At the same time step back to center and tilt your pelvis forward (pubic bone looks up).

With this wide-reaching arm movement, you take strength from the universe and guide it to your pelvis. Your weight, your center of gravity, your attention, and your breath always remain in your pelvis/genitals, even as the steps lead you alternately left and right. Stomp if the goal of the exercise is your menstruation. Tread lightly if you want to stimulate your fertility.

Note: Inhalation and exhalation take equal time in the harvest dance. This is a classic ritual dance from Africa. It may put you in a trance if you practice it too long; therefore practice with caution!

Weed note: Like the vast majority of such dances worldwide, the actual original intent of the dance *is* to induce a light trance. Trance states are not dangerous so long as they are entered into with awareness. The kinds of trances created by fertility dances make it easier to impact your reproductive choices and reproductive health. There is some evidence to indicate that so-called "primitive" peoples used such trances as a major component of fertility manipulation. Light trances strengthen the power of prayers, affirmations, and visualizations.

Chopping Wood Dance

As in the Harvest Dance, this dance helps you take energy from the heavens and direct it to your pelvis. Begin in basic fertility dance stance: knees relaxed, legs hip-distance apart, pelvis relaxed, feet parallel, arms relaxed. Breathe fully and consciously into your pelvis/genitals for one or two breaths. On an inhalation, stretch your arms upward with open hands. Lift your right leg, extend your head back, and tilt your pubic bone towards the floor (pelvis back). Your standing leg remains slightly bent.

Breathe out. Bring your right foot down, placing it parallel to the left and keeping the knees loosely flexed. Stomp if you desire to bring on your bleeding. Let your head fall forward. Make fists and bring them to your pelvis, which is now tilted forward (pubic bone up).

Breathe in and stretch up, lifting your left leg, relaxing your head back, and tilting the pubic bone down. Breathe out and stomp your left foot down (with force for menstruation, or lightly for fertility) as you bring your head forward and your clenched fists to your upthrust pelvis.

The illustration shows what the final stance of this dance looks like from the side.

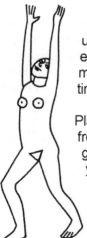

Heavenly Energy Dance

Like the previous dances, this one focuses universal healing energies on the pelvis. The expanding and contracting force of the movement makes it quite trance-inducing if done for sufficient time.

Place your legs one step apart, with the right leg in front of the left. Stretch your open hands up and gather heavenly energy while breathing in. Both your head and your pelvis are tilted back (point pubic bone down). Knees are slightly bent and feet are straight.

As you exhale, close your hands, making fists, bring your arms forward and down, and concentrate the heavenly energy into your pelvis with your fists. Let your head fall forward. Contract your pelvic muscles and point the pubic bone up. Stretch the right leg a little, but not completely.

Switch the position of your legs, so the left leg is one step in front of the right. Breathe in and reach up for heavenly energy, pointing the tailbone and the head toward each other in the back. Breathe out, pull the heavenly energy into the pelvis with the closed hands and push the pubis up toward the hands while straightening the left knee.

Be sure to breathe slowly, deeply and evenly.

Invitation Dance

Assume the basic fertility dance stance. Inhale and stretch both of your arms far forward (as if greeting or inviting someone) and, at the same time, stretch your left leg forward and up, leaving the knee bent. The other leg remains bent at the knee as well.

Exhale forcefully as you flex your left knee and draw your left leg in toward your trunk. At the same time, make fists and strongly flex your elbows. Feel strength in your entire body. Repeat, lifting your right leg forward and up as you exhale. This is a vigorous, demanding dance. It strengthens and balances, internally and externally, as it brings a powerful rush of energy into the hips and pelvis.

Breathe steadily and evenly throughout.

Embrace Dance

Inhale, spread your arms wide open to the sides, extend your head back. Keep your legs open and loose at the knees, feet parallel. Tilt your pelvis back (pubic bone tips toward the floor). Exhale; pull your head forward, round your entire back, pull your right leg up to your right breast, while your arms embrace the knee. The other leg remains bent. Tilt the pubic bone up. Still exhaling, put (or stomp) your right leg down on the floor, open your arms, throw your head back and tilt your pubic bone down. Repeat in the same way with the other leg.

Music

Music has many different effects on us and can put us in different moods. We cannot close our ears, therefore it is important to be selective about what we allow in. Electronic music or music that has been produced with synthesizers has less healing vibrations than music stemming from natural or organic instruments. For the dance phases of LUNA YOGA everybody can pick suitable music for themselves. I recommend to pick not too fast a rhythm for starters, so you won't become short of breath.

I often play "affirmations" by Kath and Ini. This is a tape produced by Australian women. They use a wide variety of instruments, including Aboriginal didjeridoos. Affirmations are invocations of positive properties that we want to support, like faith, strength, love, imagination, understanding, power, will, order, purpose, letting-go, life. The tape can be ordered from : Women's Music Collective, c/o Post Office, The Channon, New South Wales 2480, Australia.

Weed note: My choice for affirmative, woman-centered chants and music is Lisa Thiel, who has an incredible series of tapes including "Prayers for the Planet" and "Songs of the Spirit." Her tapes and an enormous variety of other wonderful music can be obtained from Ladyslipper Music, PO Box 3124R, Durham, NC 27715. For a free catalog, or to order, call 1-800-634-6044.

Pressure Points

According to the systems of acupressure and reflexology, there are certain pressure points on our bodies and feet that are reflex points for specific organs, such as the pelvic organs. These pressure points can be used to focus healing without need of direct contact with the painful area.

Whether we press these points gently or firmly, frequently or occasionally, alone or in combination with gentle sensing exercises and fertility dances, they give marked benefit. Most importantly, using them helps us improve the health and vitality of our sexual organs. The effect of the pressure points is to increase blood flow, lymphatic circulation, and energy movement into and throughout the pelvis/genitals.

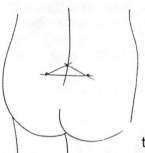

To Increase Fertility

In the flat bone of your sacrum look/feel for two dimples, one on each side. Under the dimples a small joint is hidden: the sacroiliac joint. You can massage this point gently to increase sexual intensity and pleasure. If you apply wheat germ oil to this area and rub it in well, it will greatly stimulate your fertility.

To Strengthen Bladder/Genitals

Feel below and behind the ankle bone on the inside of your foot for a tender spot. This is the pressure point that brings much energy and strength to the genitals and the urinary tract. Both gentle and strong massage have been used for relieving the pain of a bladder infection or menstrual cramps.

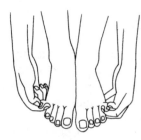

To Ease PMS & Initiate Menstruation
Bladder 67

At the far outside edge of the cuticle of the little toe is a pressure point that you may want to use when your menstruation is late, especially if you are experiencing bloatedness, distention, gas, heaviness and water retention.
Do not press this point if pregnant!!

To Heal Pelvic Problems
Gallbladder 41

Start in the web between your fourth toe and little toe. Follow this line toward the ankle until you feel a small, tender indentation. This pressure point is used to help heal many different problems of the sexual organs and urinary tract. Press with a gentle or firm pressure, as you like.

Sexual Strengthener
Bladder 60

The pressure point you'll find on the outside of your foot just behind the ankle bone is very helpful in correcting disharmonies of the pelvic organs and strengthening sexual pleasure. Easiest access is by grasping the Achilles tendon where it joins the heel and squeezing between thumb and finger.

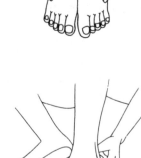

Weed note: Pressure points are easy to find; they are noticeably more tender than the surrounding tissues, especially when pressed.

Translator's note: I added the names of the corresponding acupuncture points from Traditional Chinese Medicine.

LUNA YOGA

PART FOUR

SEQUENCES

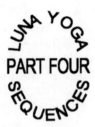

LUNA YOGA
PART FOUR
SEQUENCES

Healing Sequences

LUNA YOGA is neither a miracle cure nor an infallible technique. It works when body, mind, and spirit want to change. I think it is important to have illnesses diagnosed and to get medical advice before choosing any treatment. LUNA YOGA can be used alone; it is also a wonderful adjunct to medical treatment. It strengthens the self-healing powers, awakens the joy for life and often brings to the surface undreamed-of energies. LUNA YOGA accompanies us on our path to our inner worlds. It helps us discover our inner Wise Woman in the process, the voice of intuition, the wiseguide.

The healing sequences focus around the gentle sensing exercises from classical Hatha Yoga and fertility dances from different countries. The effect of both exercises and dances is enhanced by breathing exercises. The sensing exercises are done slowly, carefully, with deep and attentive breathing. The fertility dances are done relatively fast, dynamically, and vigorously, with rapid breaths. Pressure point massage and relaxation add the final elements for healing/health of the entire being.

I believe that LUNA YOGA is effective because it unites body, mind, and spirit and embraces the whole person. To use these sequences successfully and effectively requires that we be aware, conscious, and completely present. How easy to say this; how difficult to do! And yet, when we do, we are rewarded with serene clarity, an openess to life, increased enjoyment in all we do, and wonderfully heightened sexual pleasure. Therefore, I wish you with my full heart a delightful practice.

To Increase Fertility

Practice for no more than four days at mid-point of menstrual cycle.

- Brief relaxation for 3-5 minutes (see page 63)
- Gentle sensing exercises for 20 minutes (see p. 73)
- Breathing exercises for 5 minutes (see page 68)
- Fertility dances for 20 minutes (see page 107)
- Deep relaxation for 20 minutes (see page 63)

Optional: Pressure point massage, 5 minutes (see page 119)

In order to stimulate fertility, both partners, woman and man, need to be involved. If possible, do a short daily practice of gentle sensing exercises or any other postures that feel good to you. About twelve to fourteen days after the woman has begun her menstrual bleeding, that is, around the time of ovulation, begin this sequence.

Both partners practice the sequence daily for four consecutive days, practicing at the same time each day. It is important that the interval between the practice sessions is 24 hours.

If desired, pressure points for fertility can be added to the sequence or used instead of the breathing exercises.

Make every effort to do the twenty minutes of fertility dances without a break. It is all right if you need to dance with a light step; in this sequence the steps don't have to be executed with heavy stomping.

During and after the final deep relaxation, take care to stay warm inside and outside. Relax with a sheet or blanket over you; or, better yet, bundle up together in bed for the last relaxation. A hot water bottle is helpful unless it's summer.

If you want a drink after exercising, sip a cup of hot or warm herbal tea such as raspberry leaf, red clover, or fresh mint.

This helps preserve the warmth you have generated within your pelvis and sexual organs and encourages circulation to the reproductive area. *Avoid cold drinks. Do not bathe or take a shower*, as this will cool the reproductive fire, no matter how hot the water is.

Most of the time, ovulation will take place sometime during the four days of practice. If the woman feels this, the series can be stopped. Less than four days of this sequence is fine; but never do it for more than four days, as it is quite powerful and the generation of too much heat in the pelvis could be counter-productive.

Weed note: To increase chances of conception, the woman may wish to take 10-25 drops of wild yam tincture daily for the two-week period between menstruation and ovulation. To avoid birth defects, both partners can increase the amounts of vitamin E and folic acid in their diets. For further information on increasing fertility, see my book *Wise Woman Herbal for the Childbearing Year*.

To Induce Menstruation

Practice for no more than four days near the end of the menstrual cycle.

- Brief relaxation (see page 63)
- Sensing exercises for 20 minutes (see page 73)
- Breathing exercises for 5 minutes (see page 68)
- Fertility dances for 20 minutes (see page 107)
- Deep relaxation for 20 minutes (see page 63)

Optional: Pressure-point massage, 5 minutes (see page 119)

To induce menstruation, the woman practices this sequence for an hour a day on four consecutive days. It is important to practice daily at the same time so that every 24 hours an impulse will reach the body.

Use the most vigorous fertility dances: the ones with lots of foot stomping are best. Do not stop for any reason. Dance for the entire twenty minutes without letup.

You may do this LUNA YOGA series if you wish to avoid pregnancy, but only towards the end of your menstrual cycle, and never for more than an hour on four days in a row.

Afterwards, drink a cup of very hot ginger tea and avoid getting cold.

Weed note: Other herbs used commonly as menstrual promoters include yarrow flowers, pennyroyal herb (avoid oil), tansy flowers, and cronewort (mugwort) herb. None of these herbs used without LUNA YOGA are dependable in effecting the release of an undesired pregnancy. My book *Wise Woman Herbal for the Childbearing Year* contains a complete list of herbs used to induce menstruation and release an unwanted pregnancy.

To Alleviate Menstrual Problems

Practice daily or weekly

- Gentle sensing exercises, 20-40 minutes (see page 73)
- Breathing exercises for 5-10 minutes (see page 68)
- Pressure point massage for 5 minutes (see page 119)
- Relaxation for 5-10 minutes (see page 63)

Women who are troubled by menstrual cramping, irregular periods, premenstrual stress and bloat, recurrent vaginal and bladder infections, and other pelvic problems including ovarian cysts, will find LUNA YOGA most helpful if they practice regularly.

In all these cases, I recommend that the individual woman put together a daily exercise program of 20 to 40 minutes, consisting mostly of gentle sensing exercises. Experiment with all the exercises, so you can pick those that you really enjoy and like to do frequently. It makes no sense to torture yourself in an attempt to do something "healthy." Remember that joy is one of the most important aspects of healing.

Breathing exercises hasten the healing process, but require special attention, as they release hidden memories and because they have such a strong effect on the depth of our psyche.

Weed note: There is often a connection between sexual abuse, even indirect abuse such as advertising messages, and menstrual problems. Seek the help of a teacher, therapist, or healer/helper if need arises. Don't overdo the breathing if you are practicing daily.

Vigorous fertility dances help move and resolve memories and emotions released by breathing. As with the sensing exercises, try out several dances until you find the ones most suited to you. I recommend that dances always follow sensing exercises, whether or not you do the breathing exercises. When there are menstrual problems, limit fertility dances to no more than five minutes. After you relax deeply, drink a cup of hot tea.

Weed note: Try a cup of catnip tea or a cup of ginger tea if menstrual cramping bothers you. Try nettle or oatstraw infusion to help heal premenstrual distress. An infusion of red clover blossoms or red raspberry leaves may help women with erratic cycles. Try cornsilk tea or infusion of uva ursi to soothe and heal the bladder. Chickweed tea has been known to help dissolve cysts.

To Relieve Menopausal Distress

Practice daily or weekly

- Brief relaxation for 3-5 minutes (see page 63)
- Sensing exercises for 15-30 minutes (see page 73)
- Breathing exercises for 5-10 minutes (see page 68)
- Optional: Fertility dances for 5 minutes (see page 107)
- Pressure-point massage for 5 minutes (see page 119)
- Deep relaxation for 10 minutes (see page 63)

LUNA YOGA is an excellent method of relieving the frequency and duration of hot flashes, improving the quality and duration of sleep, preventing or correcting vaginal thinning and dryness, maintaining a healthy heart, and preventing osteoporosis. Choose any of the gentle sensing exercises and breathing exercises that feel good to you. Fertility dances can be added off and on, but don't do them daily. Pressure point massage is especially helpful in reducing emotional tension and maintaining moist, wrinkle-free skin and strong mucous membranes in the bladder and vagina.

Weed note: Try a cup of warm oatstraw infusion after your practice, or use 5-10 drops of motherwort tincture in a cup of water. For more information on relieving menopausal symptoms, see my book *Menopausal Years, the Wise Woman Way.*

To Help Heal Severe Pelvic Problems

Practice daily for an hour or more

- Brief relaxation for 2-5 minutes (see page 63)
- Sensing exercises for 40 minutes (see page 73)
- Breathing exercises for 5 minutes (see page 68)
- Pressure-point massage for 5 minutes (see page 119)
- Deep relaxation for 10-20 minutes (see page 63)

Women with severe pelvic problems such as cervical dysplasia, cervical cancer, uterine fibroids, uterine cancer, uterine hemorrhage, ovarian cancer, ovarian cysts, and extreme dysmenorrhea (menstrual pain) will find benefit, if not relief, from regular LUNA YOGA sessions, whether they choose standard medical treatments or not.

Men with severe pelvic problems such as enlarged prostate, BPH (benign prostate hypertrophy), prostate cancer, testicular cancer, and impotence will find benefit, and possibly relief from symptoms, with regular LUNA YOGA sessions, whether they choose standard medical treatments or not.

Please be aware that untreated cancer can kill.

Weed note: A recent study done at the Harvard School of Public Health showed that women who exercise regularly cut their lifetime risk of breast cancer by 35 percent and their lifetime risk of reproductuve cancers, including cervical and uterine cancers, by "an astounding" 61 percent.

To Increase Sperm Count and Quality

*Practice daily for fastest results; weekly for
slow improvement*

- Gentle sensing exercises for 15 minutes (see p. 73)
- Breathing or fertility dances for 5 minutes (see p. 68)
- Pressure point massage for 3-5 minutes (see p. 119)

A daily program of LUNA YOGA will give most men a
clearly improved sperm count and quality within three months
of practice.

Weed note: Heat destroys sperm. Hot tubs, saunas, sweat
lodges, tight jeans, and close-fitting underwear have adverse effects
on sperm production. Keeping the testicles heated to 110 degrees
Farenheit for at least thirty minutes daily for six weeks will decrease
sperm production so much, that it is virtually impossible to conceive for
the following six months. (Yes, this does work as a safe, inexpensive
form of birth control.)

Nutrition, whether poor or excellent, has a profound effect on
quantity and quality of sperm, too. Worldwide, sperm counts have
decreased by almost fifty percent in the past fifty years. Some
researchers link this with the hormone-mimicing herbicides and
pesticides that have accumulated in the world's foods during this period.
If test results show your sperm to be weak, not very mobile, and/or
insufficient for easy fertilization, you may wish to experiment with
eating organic foods, especially meats, dairy, and fats, for a period of two
to three months.

To Increase Sexual Vitality and Pleasure

For men and women; practice weekly for 60-90 minutes

- Brief relaxation for 3-5 minutes (see page 63)
- Sensing exercises for 15-30 minutes (see page 73)
- Breathing exercises for 5-10 minutes (see page 68)
- Deep relaxation for 10 minutes (see page 63)

Optional: Pressure-point massage for 5 minutes (page 119)

A regular weekly practice of LUNA YOGA is useful for men and women who wish to invigorate their sexual energy, deepen their sexual pleasure, strengthen their pelvic/reproductive organs, and circulate the healing energies of sexuality throughout their body.

The zest for life is a central subject in LUNA YOGA. The gentle sensing exercises help us focus on our sexual organs, making clear to us what immense vitality is in us. Not techniques or functions are being addressed but the origin of our life. LUNA YOGA can contribute to a deepening of our sexuality. A sensual and mindful approach to sex is the intention of many cultures and traditions.

In Tibetan Tantrism, sexual power is ritually worshipped. Yab (father) and Yum (mother) are equally necessary to preserve the earth. Through unification of both—Yab (method) and Yum (wisdom)—Buddhahood (deliverance and liberation) can be reached. Tibetan Tantra gives instruction for both: the unification of man and woman as well as the connection of male and female energies within each person.

In East Indian Hinduism the world is created through the unison of the male principle of rest and order (Shiva) with the female principle of energy and chaos (Shakti). As in Tibetan Tantrica philosophy, Hindus see the recreation of the world in every sexual act, and celebrate sexuality as the play of the goddess with the god.

Yin and Yang (female and male poles) are the pillars of our existence in Taoism. To create and recreate a balance between these poles requires lifelong mastery.

Native American philosophies see mother and father, sister and brother in everything that surrounds us. Nothing dominates the other, nothing is better than the other. Female and male are equally necessary for prosperity on earth.

Among Australian Aborigines, women and men each celebrate their own ceremonies and dream their own paths, in addition to those shared. All the rituals are equally valuable and important. Men and women unite to "dream into reality" the conception of their children.

Within a few months of undertaking regular practice of LUNA YOGA, expect to see improvement in metabolic functions (weight will decrease or increase if needed), a deep relaxation in the nervous system (with subsequent ability to carry stronger sensations of pleasure), greater health and flexibility of the pelvic organs (firmer and more sustained erections for him; multiple orgasms for her), and a greater ease in dealing with feelings (less mood swings and jealousy, heightened ability to experience intimacy).

The gentle sensing exercises can be practiced any time without restrictions, even daily if you desire. They will inevitably increase your delight and well-being. The fertility dances are enormously potent; best to limit them to times when you wish to experience the utmost in sexual pleasure.

LUNA YOGA

PART FIVE

SENSIBILITIES

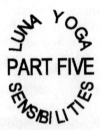

LUNA YOGA
PART FIVE
SENSIBILITIES

Something Sensible
and Something Sensuous
for our Senses

LUNA YOGA is a holistic way of healing which enriches our lives, enhances our sensuousness, and helps us become more sensitive to ourselves and others.

Can we be sensitive, sensual, and sensible, too? I want to end the separation that ascribes sensibility to men and sensuality to women. We can have it all! When we practice LUNA YOGA we experience stimulation as well as relaxation, movement as well as rest. We learn to honor our individual needs, our own changeable natures. Then we find that sensible and sensuous can co-exist happily and easily.

With the aid of Water, Air, Fire, and Earth, we can add to the basics of LUNA YOGA. Here are a few of my favorite ways to do this. I trust that you will experiment sensibly and find what feels sensual and good to you. Take your courage in hand and modify my suggestions to your own taste. Let your own sense of well-being decide.

Water

Water is the element associated with the female. Softly flowing it adapts to any shape. We connect emotions with the water, especially tears and grief, as emotions move us. Water helps us forget and forgive. Water is so necessary for our survival. Water is so strong and so gentle at the same time. Living beings consist mostly of water .

Kidney and Bladder regulate the water balance in our body. The direction for water is traditionally the West, from which most of the rain clouds approach us, in Europe. Cancer, Scorpio, and Pisces are the astrological signs for the water element. "Steady drop hollows the stone" is a German saying that teaches us about the soft power of water.

Herbal Teas

Herbal teas are wonderful drinks summer or winter. After completing a LUNA YOGA series, I suggest a cup of hot herbal tea. It supports the processes that have been initiated through the movements, and preserves the warmth within the pelvis.

I don't always drink the same teas; I like diversity. I don't want to become habituated or have less effect from the herb.

Unless otherwise indicated, I use one teaspoon of herbs per cup of tea, pour boiling water on the mixture, and let it steep for five to ten minutes.

Drink an amount that corresponds to your thirst. For teas which also have an effect on Liver and Gallbladder four cups a day should be the maximum.

Here's some favorite tea blends from my home, Hessia.
To Your Health!

Weed note: Unlike black tea and coffee, nourishing and tonifying herbs such as Raspberry leaf, Nettle leaf, Motherwort, and Lemon Balm are as safe as carrots and spinach. And, like any food, these herbs may be used day after day with no habituation and no loss of effect.

For maximum nourishment and effect from your herbs, try an infusion instead of a tea. I use a huge handful of dried herb (up to a full ounce) in a quart jar, which I then fill to the top with boiling water and tightly lid. I let it steep, undisturbed, for 4-6 hours. The resulting brew is dark and rich and can be drunk iced or heated up. Strain and refrigerate after opening jar.

Sweet Dreams Tea

3 parts Marjoram herb (*Origanum marjorana*)
3 parts Spearmint herb (*Mentha spicata*)
2 parts Dandelion leaves or root (*Taraxacum off.*)
2 parts Stinging Nettle leaves (*Urtica dioica*)
1 part Calendula flowers (*Calendula off.*)
1 part Bachelor's Button/Cornflowers (*Centaurea cyanus*)
1/2 part Rose Blossoms (*Rosa sp.*)
1/2 part Orange Blossoms (*Citrus sinensis*)
pinch of Rue (*Ruta graveolens*)

This tea has a healing effect on the pelvic organs. It encourages energy flow to the uterus and helps relieve uterine tension and menstrual cramps. It is a good drink before bedtime and will bring you deep dreams.

Weed note: This originally contained 3 parts Rue, but I do not feel that it is safe for most women to use Rue in such quantity. CAUTION: Rue is considered an abortifacient herb. DO NOT USE RUE if you are pregnant, trying to get pregnant, or contemplating pregnancy in the near future. This makes a wonderful infusion if you omit the Rue.

Strong Dreams Tea

2 parts Lemon Thyme herb (*Thymus sp.*)
2 parts Stinging Nettle herb (*Urtica dioica*)
2 parts Dandelion herb or root (*Taraxacum off.*)
1 part Calendula flowers (*Calendula off.*)
1 part Bee Balm herb (*Monarda didyma*)
1 part Strawberry leaf (*Fragaria sp.*)
1 part Mugwort/Cronewort herb (*Artemisia vulgaris*)

This tea aids digestion, strengthens the kidneys, improves the blood, and stimulates the flow of bile. It is especially helpful for women with PMS. Try a cup and see if it isn't wonderful for a healing sleep with potent dreams. I also use it as a support for a course of homeopathic treatment.

Weed note: For psychedelic dreams, try this as an infusion.

Tea to Ease Light Menstrual Cramps

3 parts of Lady's Mantle herb (*Alchemilla vulgaris*)
2 parts Yarrow flowers (*Achillea millefolium*)
2 parts German Chamomile flowers (*Matricaria chamomilla*)
1 part Garden Thyme herb (*Thymus vulgaris*)
1 part Wild Thyme (Quendal) herb (*Thymus serpyllum*)

Use a full tablespoon of this mix in one cup of boiling water; steep for 15 minutes. For women who usually cramp when bleeding, begin drinking this tea at least four days before you expect your menstruation, a cup in the morning and a cup at night, and continue until you have stopped bleeding. This tea is a strong diuretic and eliminates held water, making it helpful in relieving PMS problems. I especially recommend this tea for girls in puberty and those just starting to menstruate. I love its soothing cramp relief.

Tea to Ease Strong Menstrual Cramps

3 parts St.John's/Joan's Wort flowers (*Hypericum perforatum*)
3 parts German Chamomile flowers (*Matricaria chamomilla*)
2 parts Hops flowers (*Humulus lupulus*)
2 part Woodruff herb (*Asperula odorata*)
2 parts Lady's Mantle herb (*Alchemilla vulgaris*)
1 part Motherwort herb (*Leonurus cardiaca*)

Use 1 tablespoon herbs per cup; steep at least 15 minutes. I have used this reliable combination with success for women who bleed for a long time, and for women who have very strong menstrual cramps. I also think of it as excellent for women before, during, and after menopause.

Weed note: This combination is especially powerful brewed as an infusion rather than a tea. Or, for ease, use 25 drops tincture of St. Joan's Wort, 15 drops tincture of Lady's Mantle, and 10 drops Motherwort tincture in a cup of Chamomile tea.

Deep Dreams Tea

1 part Peppermint herb (*Mentha piperata*)
1 part Marjoram herb (*Origanum marjorana*)
pinch of Rue (*Ruta graveolens*)

This tea is said to promote healthy sleep and to nourish and support the functioning of the sexual organs. I find it helpful for women with gynecological problems.

Weed note: The original recipe called for an equal part of Rue herb. See warnings on Rue in recipe for Sweet Dreams Tea. DO NOT drink more than one cup of this tea a day for any reason. DO NOT infuse, use only as a tea.

Tea to Aid Menstruation

4 parts Lemon Balm herb (*Melissa off.*)
3 parts Hops flowers (*Humulus lupulus*)
3 parts German Chamomile flowers (*Matricaria chamomilla*)
2 parts Rosemary herb (*Rosmarinus off.*)
2 parts Fennel seeds (*Foeniculum vulgare*)
1 part Stinging Nettle herb (*Urtica dioica*)

I use two teaspoons of this mix in a cup of boiling water and let it steep for 15 minutes. Starting about a week before my menses are due, I drink two cups daily in the morning and the late afternoon. This tea helps me ease into bleeding. It is especially recommended for women of any age who are struggling with worries, fright, restlessness, sorrow, and overburden, as well as nervous excitement. I find it calms me down and cheers me up.

Weed note: This one would also be fantastic at infusion strength.

Spicy Dreams Tea

1 part Cinnamon Stick (*Cinnamomum sp*)
1 part Ginger Root (*Zingiber off.*)
1 part Vanilla Bean
1 part Licorice Root (*Glycyrrhiza glabra*)
1 part Marshmallow Root (*Althaea off.*)
5 seed pods of Cardamom (*Elettaria cardamomum*)

I use a thumbnail-sized piece of each herb in a quart of water, simmered for about 15 minutes as an aphrodisiac. Complete with milk and honey, it stimulates libido.

Tea to Stimulate Menstruation

Ingredients for part A
1 teaspoon Groundsel (*Senecio vulgaris*) leaves
1 teaspoon Shepherd's Purse (*Capsella bursa-pastoris*) herb
Mix dried herbs together; steep in 1 cup boiling water for 15 minutes.

Weed notes: If neither fresh nor dried herbs are available, use 10 drops of each tincture instead.

Ingredients for part B
2 teaspoons Horsetail herb (*Equisetum arvense*)
Let soak in one cup of cold water for an hour, and then bring to a quick boil.

Procedure for preparation
Mix A and B together or drink singly, two cups daily before the onset of menstruation. This tea is good for both men and women during mid-life crisis.

Weed note: American herbalists are less familiar with the power of Senecios than European herb women, who use the Senecios frequently. I've come to love these so-called dangerous plants for their ability to increase energy in women's reproductive/genital area (many women report aphrodisiac effects from daily use of 5 drops), to normalize erratic hormones, and to help women who have extremely painful periods.

As given, this formula is not abortifacient, nor even emmenagogic; it is exceedingly unlikely that its use would disrupt an early pregnancy or even truly stimulate menses to come before their time. It could help prevent heavy bleeding in women with fibroids or endometriosis and regular use would certainly reduce and hopefully prevent even the most severe menstrual cramping.

Senecios do have the ability to increase energy to the uterine area so dramatically that birth and bleeding are hastened. Instead of making two teas, I would use 10 drops of tincture of fresh Liferoot (*Senecio aureus*) flowers and 10 drops of tincture of fresh Shepherd's Purse herb in a cup of Horsetail tea, and take it every three to four hours, for up to five days.

Vitality Tea

1 part Turmeric root (*Curcuma longa*)
1 part Cinnamon bark (*Cinnamomum sp.*)
1 part fresh Ginger root (*Zingiber off.*)
4 seed pods of Cardamom (*Elettaria cardamomum*)
1 part Caraway (or Cumin) seeds (*Carum carvi*)
1/2 part Cloves (*Syzigium aromaticum*)
1/2 part Anise (or Fennel) seeds (*Pimpinella anisum*)

I cut pieces of Turmeric, Cinnamon and Ginger the size of my thumbnail and simmer them in one quart of water for a few minutes. Then I add the Cardamom pods and boil for another short while. Lastly, I add the Cloves and aromatic seeds. bring them to a quick boil, turn off the heat and strain the drink into a quart jar containing a few leaves of Peppermint, where it steeps a few minutes more.

Drink this tea only in day time, as it is very stimulating for all metabolic processes.

Calming Tea

1 part Raspberry leaf (*Rubus* species)
1 part Lemon Balm herb (*Melissa off.*)
1 part Chamomile blossoms (*Matricaria chamomilla*)

Steep 1 tablespoon of herbs in 2 to 4 cups boiling water for five minutes.

This tea mix is calming to the nerves, relaxing for the muscles and nourishing for the pelvic organs. What a warm and cozy brew! After drinking it, you will find yourself warmed, your blood circulation improved and your lower abdomen radiating a sensation of comfort and ease.

Aviva Steiner's Relaxing Tea

1 part Orange blossoms (*Citrus sinensis*)
1 part Rose petals (*Rosa sp.*)
1 part Passion Flower herb/blossoms (*Passiflora incarnata*)
  optional: 1 part Peony (*Paeonia off.*) flowers

Steep 1 tablespoon in 2-4 cups boiling water for up to 10 minutes. Drink in the evening to ensure a deep and satisfying sleep. It relaxes the pelvic organs and prepares us for fertility.

Summertime Tea

1 part Lemongrass herb (*Cymbopogon citratus*)
1 part Lemon Thyme herb (*Thymus* x *citriodorus*)
1 part Vervain flowering herb (*Verbena off.*)

Steep 1 tablespoon in 2 to 4 cups boiling water for 5 minutes. Very refreshing when days grow long. Delicious and enlivening, hot or cold. Try with honey for a special treat.

Wintertime Tea

1 Cinnamon Stick
1 handful Linden Flowers (*Tillia sp.*)
1 piece Ginger Root (size of a thumbnail), finely chopped

Steep all three herbs in 3 cups of boiling water for 15 to 20 minutes.   This tea warms body, mind, and soul.

Weed note: Linden blossoms are a fabled cold preventative. Ginger root is prized for its ability to warm the abdomen. Cinnamon is warming and aids good blood circulation. A handsome trio to take to bed on a chilly winter evening.

Women's Tea

1 part Raspberry leaves (*Rubus ideaus*)
1 part Yarrow flowers (*Achillea millefolium*)
1 part Lady's Mantle herb (*Alchemilla vulgaris*)
1 part Strawberry leaves (*Fragaria sp.*)
1 part Blackberry leaves (*Rubus villosus*)

Pour 3 cups of boiling water over 1 tablespoon herbs; steep for 10 minutes. This tea strengthens and nourishes the female reproductive tract and harmonizes the sexual organs.

Weed note: Brew to infusion strength; drink two cups a day and prepare to experience the energy of your womb as you never have before. OK to leave out Blackberry and/or Strawberry leaves.

Moon Tea

2 parts Queen of the Meadow leaves (*Eupatorium purpurea*)
2 parts Chicory leaves (*Cichorium intybus*)
1 part Bee Balm flowers (*Monarda didyma*)
1 part Calendula flowers (*Calendula off.*)
1 part Cornflower blossoms (*Centaurea cyanus*)

Add 1 tablespoon herbs to 4 cups boiling water; steep for 10 minutes. I drink this wonderful tea at the full and new moon. It supports the influence of the moon, thus it is "for the heart," but it contains far more virtues and powers, which you will discover as you use it. I find it especially effective when I want to manifest my creativity in material form; this tea helps me bring my ideas to the outside. May the heart of LUNA YOGA touch your heart in this brew.

May you benefit from these teas.

Bath Mixtures

Baths combine well with LUNA YOGA if taken *before* your practice. Don't bathe or shower for at least eight hours after your LUNA YOGA sessions as the water will take away the warmth you've worked hard to generate in your body and your pelvis. Bathing or showering after your sessions also washes away your skin resistance and the fine protective moisture film that is formed on your skin during LUNA YOGA exercises. So, if you practice in the morning, don't entrust yourself to the wet element until the evening; if LUNA YOGA is your evening activity, don't apply water until the next morning.

A bath *before* your practice session loosens and relaxes your muscles, allowing you to assume many positions with greater ease. Take sufficient time for your bath so you can really enjoy it.

Here are a few of my favorite herbal bath recipes. May they inspire courage for your own creations.

Rejuvenating Salt Water Bath

Depending on the size of your bathtub, dissolve 2 to 4 pounds of salt in hot water. It is best to use sea-salt, but rock-salt will do as well. Choose the temperature to your liking, relinquish yourself to the bath for up to 20 minutes, and then rest well. Be careful: a salt water bath creates sweating and has a strong effect on the circulation.

Weed note: Kosher salt is excellent in this kind of bath, as is seaweed. In fact, there are even special seaweeds sold to scrub yourself with, thus giving you double benefits.

Relaxing Blossom Bath

Fill a small cloth bag with flower blossoms such as Orange blossoms, Rose petals, Passion Flowers, and Jasmine Blossoms. Hang it in your bathwater and the flowers will emanate a pleasant, delicate scent that will relax all your tensions.

Buttermilk Bath

If you tend toward dry skin, or dry vaginal tissues, add 3 to 5 quarts of buttermilk to your bathtub and relish a luxurious warm white bath.

Weed notes: A yogurt bath is even better. This one dates back to Cleopatra's day, and does it ever work wonders for dry tissues.

Heublumen Bath to Stimulate Menstrual Flow

Put two to three handfuls of Heublumen into a cloth bag and float it in the bathtub, partially filled with hot water. Add yourself to the bath; bring up the temperature carefully and slowly. To improve the effect, do a deep relaxation afterwards.

Weed note: Heublumen are hay blossoms. Hay is grass. You can use any grass flowers for this bath. Or you can use Oatstraw. Oatstraw baths are a classical remedy for those with jangled nerves. This bath will not induce abortion.

Moonwater

Moonwater strengthens female power, whether used by men or women.

The art of preparing Moonwater is ancient; its origins are lost to the darkness of matriarchal history. But the recipe is simple, and as easily done today as by any women who lived thousands of years ago.

Begin by making a careful choice of your container, which could be the same for all the different signs and phases of the moon, or which could vary as the moon does—sometimes large and sometimes small, sometimes bright and sometimes dark. You might even have twelve different ones corresponding to the astrological signs.

Your container needs to be able to hold as much water as you would use up in a month, drinking one sip a day. And, you need to be able to close it tightly, so your moonwater won't evaporate.

On the eve of the full moon, fill the container with fresh water. If you like, add a piece of jewelry or a stone that corresponds to the moon's sign. (I don't have any rules for this, but freely associate what the different signs symbolize.) During the full moon, the moon's sign is opposite the Sun's sign.

Expose your filled container to the full moon for the entire night. Place it outside and in the open where the full moon can shine into it for as many hours as possible. Next morning, take your first sip of moon water. This water that has gathered the moon's energy will be the first thing we consume every day from now until the next full moon. Each morning, on an empty stomach, one more sip is consumed, and we strengthen ourselves with the properties of full moon: creativity, abandon, imagination, wildness, strength, brightness.

I wish you much joy with the water of the moon!

Moon Days

In classical Yoga there is a tradition of special moon days. I suspect this is a remnant from the matriarchal origins of Yoga.

The most attention is paid to the days/nights of the full and new moons. It is said that the moon's power of attraction and repulsion can be utilized to harmonize the human metabolism on these particular days.

In addition, there is the eleventh day after the full moon, and the eleventh day after the new moon. On these days—called Ekadasi—the moon has a specific angle to the earth that can be used to create a beneficial influence on our body fluids and their movements.

Strict yogis and yoginis focus completely on the moon for these four days out of each month. They don't eat or drink, they meditate, maintain silence, and are completely centered on the moon.

For our modern lives, without the support of an ashram, we need to modify these strict rules. What feels good to you? Is this an especially good time to do LUNA YOGA? Or a time to rest from it? Perhaps you will want to eat lightly on the days of full moon and new moon? or to drink only herbal teas? Can you find time to do a special meditation on these four days? Pay attention to your talking. Does it need to be said? What is it like to be silent?

Weed note: Modern-day moon days are the four consecutive days of a woman's menstrual period. Many women find that their menstrual and premenstrual problems greatly diminish when they take moon days: time to be alone, time to be in silence, time to be in nature, time to bleed, time to flow, time to just be. Post-menopausal women will no doubt benefit from using the moon days described by Adelheid as a way to continue to keep in contact with the moon, their LUNA YOGA, their wombs, and the springs of their deep inner knowing.

Air

Air, the element connected with spirit, the mind, the intellect, thinking. Clear air of pure reason. Winds that change and renew. Breezes and cold fronts that puff through us. Storms and hurricanes that rage and create havoc. Air can caress us; it is essential for our life; we are constantly connected with it through our breath. In astrology the signs of Gemini, Libra, and Aquarius embody the airy element. The lungs are the organ of air. Air's direction is the East: sunrise, morning, spring. To some Native Americans, air symbolizes exchange and partaking in creativity. Air is not palpable. Air cannot be seized. Air is free, without form. The imagination is at home in the air element. Laughter and mirth belong to air, as do easiness and heart's desire.

Meditation

Meditation is rooted linguistically in Latin, *in medium ire*, to find one's own center, to go to the center, or to get to the bottom of the matter. In meditation we go to the center of our own being.

Meditation can help us discover the inner quiet that comes when we accept ourselves as we are, and slide free from our old patterns of denial. Meditation can help us recognize our truth. I encourage couples who want to conceive to meditate with their wish and listen carefully to the inner voices they find in meditation, and thus to discover hidden truths.

Meditation can help us be aware and alive, everywhere and any time—even (especially!) in daily life. In Japanese Zen Buddhism, we learn that every act can be done in meditation. The same idea has been passed down by the European mystics. East Indian Karma Yoga teaches that everything should arise from an inner attitude of devotion, and that doing and non-doing should be conscious.

Whatever we do, if we do it from the depths of our heart and with total focus, we will be true to ourselves. Meditation opens us to the depths of our hearts and teaches us how to focus. Meditation is a beautiful way to create a ritual of retreat into our selves.

This retreat into our own natures in turn awakens us to the outside. Meditation does not mean escape from the world. Meditation in LUNA YOGA is to help us open to our surroundings. In meditation, I stay aware and attentive to myself and develop the same awareness and attention toward my environment. LUNA YOGA meditation opens the inner world and creates an expanded access to success and happiness in the outer world as well.

LUNA YOGA meditation is strengthened by the powers of the moon. The moon helps us make ourselves ready for change. The moon helps us find acceptance of cycles and rhythms. The moon helps us let go of old concepts; she creates space for new energies. Like the moon passing through her phases, we understand that to renew ourselves, we must nourish what needs to mature to its fullness and perfection, then let go of it. We are always developing and unfolding, becoming, growing.

"Open space—nothing sacred." That is how the late British-American meditation teacher Alan Watts referred to meditation, from which, it is said, arises true clarity, serenity, and calmness.

Begin by meditating alone. This helps you stay more in your own center. When we meditate in a group the joint energy grows. Meditation is not something that you do; it is something that involves you. And that means that you get involved with yourself. Meditation is an exciting adventure.

Meditation does not require a lot of preparation. You'll need:

- A quiet place, in the house or outside.
- Some time, in which you are not rushed or interrupted. The times of transition from day to night and from night to day, dawn and dusk, are said to be especially conducive times for meditation. Also the energies of the full moon and new moon help us deepen our meditation.
- A cushion or mat or other aid to sitting in a posture that is comfortable to you. (OK to sit on a chair, stool, or couch.) If you can sit well on the ground, make yourself comfortable there. That does not mean that you should let yourself slouch. On the contrary, you should sit in a way that your breath can flow freely and your back can be held upright with least effort, so it won't be too hard to sit still for 15 to 30 minutes.

That's all.

Breathing Meditation

Focus on the flow of your own breath. Again and again, return to your breath. Give it your full awareness. Let your breath come and go like waves in the sea. If thoughts emerge, let them pass by and gently bring the focus back to your breath. Just stay with your breath—nothing else.

Taming the Monkeys

The image of wild monkeys is common in South Indian writings on meditation. They are a symbol for thoughts, which move constantly like monkeys in the jungle, disturbing our peace and serenity. If we want be vital and aware, we have to quiet down our thoughts. When we simply watch our thoughts, their comings and goings, instead of trying to switch them off, then they calm down. In this meditation don't hold onto a thought, don't follow a thought, simply let them go.

Eventually you will notice pauses in which you are, indeed, free from whirling thoughts. Aha! You have tamed the monkeys.

To Take Yourself Seriously and to be Amused by It

An old Ceylonese monk warmly recommended this delightful meditation to me. Sit quietly and comfortably. Sense whatever is happening: your nose is itching, your finger wants to be scratched, your legs fall asleep. You don't *do* anything. You simply perceive what is happening; you notice, with wonder, your own distractions; you allow your sensations without intervention. The more you can let go, the less you will be bound to agitated feelings. The deeper within we reach to touch ourselves with love, the greater a sense of peace we feel in our being.

Tratak

This is a light and fire meditation. It is said to strengthen and benefit the eyes.

Take a candle, light the wick, and place it before your eyes so that you can look at it comfortably. The flame should be eye-level. Start by blinking your eyes a few times very quickly, then slower and finally close your eyes for a moment to relax them. Then open your eyes again and look with a soft gaze and without blinking into the candle flame. Do that till you feel a tingle and tearing in your eyes. Then close your eyes again and probably the image of the candle flame will appear before your inner vision. Don't forget to breathe deeply yet softly; don't hold your breath in all that concentration.

OM Meditation

The Sanskrit syllable OM is said to be the primordial sound of humanity. It is especially beneficial for meditation. Similar sounds occur in all cultures and languages and are often used in sacred ceremonies. Just think of the completion of Christian prayers with an "Amen." In Jewish or Muslim prayer houses it resounds as "amain."

OM is the sound-image of the frequency which connects us with universal power. The old yogic writings claim that this frequency can harmonize the functioning of every cell, because it contains not only the frequency of the earth, but the entire universe. The music scholar Joachim Ernst Behrendt writes that OM reflects the frequency of the Earth. OM is said to be healing to the frequencies of human energy, calming and restorative to all beings.

The sound OM recreates the world anew, says tradition. OM is the symbol and sound of creation.

Meditate on OM by imagining the sound, let the tone sound inside you. Or chant OM as you breathe out. Return your focus, again and again, back to OM. If your thoughts wander, come back to OM.

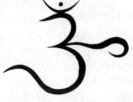

OM: The lower curve is longer and represents the dream state, the upper curve stands for the waking state, and the curve emerging from the center symbolizes the dreamless deep sleep state. The crescent above stands for Maya, the veil of illusion, and the dot above it for transcendence.

When the individual is able to step through the veil of unconsciousness and delusion, and stay focused in the one-pointedness of transcendence, then s/he will experience freedom from the three states of illusion: waking, dreaming, and sleeping.

Dream Journeys

Whatever moves us within, may it be thoughts or emotions, has outer expressions, causes, repercussions. We become what we think and feel. However we view the world, that is the way it will appear to us. Dreams can help us alter our view. Dream journeys offer a chance to explore actively our inner world and try out new patterns of behavior. This applies to both the journeys of our daydreams and the dreams in our night sleep.

What we experience during the day emerges at night transformed in our dreams. What impresses us wants to be expressed. We don't need to leave this interplay of outside and inside to chance. We can interfere in a creative way. Before falling asleep, make a resolution to dream about something or someone specific. Take anything that occupies your thoughts into your dreams and seek understanding, even answers, there. In dreams, our unconscious and our subconscious are free to tell us the answers for which we have long been waiting.

Conscious-centered daydreaming is another way to uncover answers from the depths of our selves. For this, seek out a beautiful place outside or inside, where you can relax undisturbed. Make yourself completely comfortable and pleasant in a lying or sitting pose in which you can let go comfortably.

Concentrate on yourself, close your eyes, let your breath become quiet and clear, and set up a way to protect or guard yourself. This is important, because you want to open yourself for the influences of other planes. So imagine something that will protect you. That could be a circle of light, a stone circle, or you could light candles or incense sticks. To feel protected is what counts.

Then just let go and tune in to your theme, let thoughts

and emotions come, images and sounds, sensations and memories. Don't judge or interfere, just observe what wants to reveal itself.

Some kinds of daydreams are more controlled than this. These controlled daydreams are called journeys, or shamanic journeys, or trances, or even guided meditations. We can go on such "journeys" alone or with others, guided by an outer voice, a tape recording, or our inner voice. As for all journeys, good preparation is recommended, an open heart to take in all the adventures—and rest to muse about and process the experiences.

I am offering myself as a travel guide, to give you a taste of some of the journeys I've taken, some of the places I've visited. I hope to inspire you to explore new continents for yourself. The maps of our inner worlds still have many blank spots.

Here are a few more possible "itineraries": A journey to the "Wise Healer Within" could lead you to your inner organs, to the depths of your body and being, to awaken your self-healing powers. A journey to "My Place of Power" offers an opportunity to explore one's own specific places of power. If you undertake a journey "Through the Seasons," you will connect yourself to the cycles of nature. There are no limits to the journeys you can take to the realms of your imagination. If you want inspiration for dream journeys, I highly recommend Diane Mariechild's book *Mother Wit*.

The duration of the journey depends on your own sense of time. But take into account that the seduction of a muse requires leisurely kisses. My dream journeys last from a half hour to a full hour. That includes preparation, tuning in, relaxation, centering and guarding, and then the journey itself. Finally I give myself time to integrate the treasures from the depths of my unconscious into my consciousness, by writing down the experiences of my journey, or by drawing them, or by sharing them with someone.

The Red Journey

Prepare yourself and your space so you feel safe and calm. Relax, center and protect yourself. Let your breath become quiet and regular, be completely with yourself. Feel your body, notice your heartbeat and your pulse, and let yourself be carried by your blood streaming through your veins to your genitals.

Notice how your pelvis and sexual organs feel. What do you sense? Are there words, memories, colors, sensations? What is happening inside of you at this moment? How does it feel? Stay with these impressions and sensations. They are true. They are part of your uniqueness. Take time to listen to the inner truths of your own genitals.

Then ask your womb, your pelvis, your vagina to remember your first menstruation. What was your emotional experience? Did you know about it before it happened? Who told you about it and how? What was your physical experience? Were you in pain? Was there a lot of blood? Did you bleed on your clothes?

Deep in the cave of your memory lies the shining stone of this sacred time in your life: your transformation from maiden to woman-who-bleeds. Trace this experience, however it might have been, and know that you can change it, right now, if you wish. You can decide how you want to experience menstruation, no matter what your first messages were. If your memories of menstruation are unpleasant, you are now free to decide how it will be in the future and to what extent you wish to be influenced by the past.

Let arise before your inner eye a menstruation during which you felt especially well. What was that day like for you? What did you like about it? Why did the beautiful memory stay with you? What can you learn from this experience? What steps can you take to create more experiences of menstruation that are beautiful, pain-free, and good for you?

Let your imagination become very active. How do you want to experience your menstrual periods? How would you create it if you could have it exactly as you desire? You deserve to experience menstruation as a time of power, not pain; as a time of vision, not craziness; as a time of beauty, not something to be dreaded. You deserve whatever you need. Let your imagination's inner pictures become so vivid that they are more real than reality.

When you are done, stretch, open your eyes, and return fresh and relaxed into the present time and your usual sense of self and space.

Journey to the Four Elements

Give yourself time and space to be alone, without disruption, for at least thirty minutes. Center, breathe, protect yourself, and relax deeply and completely. Dive deep into the depths of your being and ask for the way to the elementals to be opened. This journey will lead to the four elements of our existence. Earth. Air. Water. Fire. But it is really a journey of exploration of your Self.

Call upon the presence of the Earth, the Earth who carries you. What does that mean to you? What does Earth mean to you? What do you want to entrust to the Earth? What do you ask from her? What does Earth give you? Take time to ponder these questions and listen long enough for the answers. Earth is rather slow by human standards. The Earth is associated with melancholic temperaments.

Call upon the presence of the Air, the Air which is quick and moving. What does Air carry toward you? What do you experience through Air? What do you give to Air? And what does Air give to you? Allow enough time for your exchange with the vital air, though her answers will come quickly. Air is associated with sanguine temperaments.

Call upon the presence of the Water, the Water which is flowing, slow or fast, the Water which constantly adjusts its shape. What does Water mean to you? What message does Water carry for you? And what do you give Water as she goes on her way? Listen carefully to the many voices of water. Water is associated with phlegmatic temperaments.

Wild Fire is blazing, burning, showing itself. Call upon the presence of Fire. What do you have in common with Fire? Where do you need Fire? What can Fire convey to you? What do you entrust to Fire? What does Fire mean to you? Give Fire enough time to communicate clearly. Fire is associated with choleric temperaments.

The elements can transform for us all that we have outgrown. They liberate us from the burden of carrying our past mistakes, our past grievances, our past pains, our past frustrations. Each element offers us a special way to change; each offers an opportunity to become more clear. Give to the different elements whatever you want to transform into new strength, new growth, new understanding, new pleasure. Accept from them solidity, imagination, ease, energy.

When you have completed the process of exchanging energy between yourself and the elements, stretch, open your eyes, and return to your familiar world. You'll find you are relaxed and filled with new vitality.

Chakra Journey

Chakra is a Sanskrit word that means "circle, vortex, eddy, or wheel." Thus, the circling, wheeling, energy fields in our bodies have come to be known as chakras.

The chakras cannot be found in a physical examination of the body, though they are associated or paired with physical nerve plexuses and endocrine glands. (Most cultures have some concept of chakras: in Traditional Chinese Medicine, they are acupuncture points; in Christian art, they become halos.)

A journey to your chakras can have many effects: it can be relaxing, it can help you untie old entanglements, it can charge you with powerful life energy, it can vastly increase the healing potential of your body, it can create a harmonizing effect on all your vital functions.

Since so much can be received from a visit to any one chakra, it is well to do this journey several times. Let us give our full attention and awareness to the journey to the chakras, visiting just one or two at a time. Only if you have pressing need, or a full day of uninterrupted time and leisure, would you want to visit all seven energy fields in one journey.

Relax, breathe, and guard yourself. Sink into your inner self. Be completely present with yourself. Feel sheltered and one with the universe. Imagine your body precisely and relax from your feet to your head. Now bring your attention to your spine. Breathe deeply, in and out, and feel how the air of your breath is gliding along your spine.

Breathe into the very base of your spine. This is the first chakra, *Muladhara* in Sanskrit, the **root chakra**, at the coccyx. It is your basic foundation; it connects you with the earth. This chakra regulates elimination processes. Its color is dark red.

Breathe into the dark red root chakra. The sense of smell unfolds here. Eating, drinking and sleeping are at home here.

In this chakra an understanding for right behavior in the world is developed. Here we can be safe enough to experience and love our fears and insecurities. Here ego develops into identity. Growth begins here. Knowledge about the divinity of humanness is rooted here.

Breathe in and out of the root chakra for a while: What vibrations predominate? Release those you no longer need or want. Are there discordant vibrations? Imagine a dark red color radiating powerfully and evenly from your root chakra.

Breathe into the top of the pubic bone or the sacrum. This is the second chakra, *Swadhisthana* in Sanskrit, the **sacral chakra** or seat of self, located near our sexual glands. It includes the digestive system and the genitals. Its color is orange.

Breathe into the orange sacral chakra. Here taste and emotions are at home. The element water and relationships to other people are associated with it. We learn the use of our creative energies in this chakra: procreation, conception, wisdom about the preservation of the world.

Breathe in and out of the sacral chakra. Sensuality, sexuality, significance are the key words for this energy center. What vibrations are in your Swadhisthana chakra? You are now free to let go of the ballast and regenerate yourself. Let the color red stream through you.

Breathe into the center of your navel. This is the third chakra, *Manipura* in Sanskrit, the **solar plexus chakra**, center of inner power, the inner sun. It includes the liver, gall bladder, stomach, pancreas and kidneys. The solar plexus shines yellow. It relates to the eyes, to seeing, and to fire.

Weed Note: In traditional Chinese medicine, the eyes are the opening to the liver.

Breathe into the solar plexus fire. Allow it to purify you, to show you the truth of yourself. Use it to strengthen your ability to act from your own center, especially in your relationships to others. Feel its power. Power is only what we make of it. Here is the wisdom to learn to use power appropriately.

Breathe in and out of your solar plexus. Feel the vibrations residing there. Utilize the clarifying power of fire to burn away attachments that you no longer need and let your navel center radiate in renewed freshness.

Breathe into the center of your chest. This is the fourth or center chakra, *Anahata* in Sanskrit, the **heart chakra**. It includes the lungs as well as the heart. Its color is green and healing. It opens us to heartfelt love and compassion for others.

Breathe into the green heart chakra. Feel the colorless, shapeless air as it enters your lungs, your body. Let it nourish your wisdom and inner strength, your intuition and your tenderness. As you breathe, let your desires and cravings fall away. Let the love you've been given enter you fully and cut all the strings that were attached to it.

Breathe in and out of your heart chakra. Let your heart speak and listen carefully. What is vibrating in your heart center? Can you dare to love yourself? Trust that the universe will love you? Do you believe that you must be dependent to get love from others? The culture tells women that. But true independence always attracts love from others. When you find your own heart, your own source of inspiration, you emanate an energy which is calm, peaceful, heartfelt, and incredibly exciting.

Breathe into the center of your throat. This is the fifth chakra, *Vishuddha* in Sanskrit, the **throat chakra**. It includes the thyroid gland and affects the ears and listening, the voice, sounds, the mouth. Its color is blue-violet.

Breathe into the blue throat chakra. Feel the vibrations of all the sounds around you. Make soft or loud sounds. Let your intuition guide you into wordless realms of understanding.

Hum or moan or growl or purr. Let your senses and emotions flow on the tides of sound and follow the path of your own inner wisdom. Offer your pain sympathy and compassion.

Breathe in and out of the throat chakra. What chokes your voice? When do you deny your truth? Who wouldn't listen to you? Release and reject those things that strangle you. What supports your truth? Who validates your reality? Where do you feel safe to speak freely? Nourish and cherish the vibrations that support your story, your song, your words.

Breathe into the point between the eyebrows (and a little above). This is the sixth chakra, *Ajna* in Sanskrit, the **third eye,** master point of consciousness. Golden light emanates from the third eye when it is fully open. It includes the pituitary gland, the primary control organ of the endocrine system.

Breathe into the gold-tinged darkness behind the third eye. Here seeing and perception are sheltered. Here we can learn to recognize the many forms and expressions of our ever-changing self. Here we can see, with a shock of recognition, our own past, every apect of our present, and our multiple futures. The third eye sees with the clarity of crystal, if we truly desire it, but I advise you to be cautious with this gift.

Breathe in and out of the third eye chakra and sense the vibrations that gather there. Which sustain your vision? Which cloud your sight? Release any ties that keep your eyes closed to your true beauty and uniqueness.

Breathe into the very top point of the head. This is the seventh and final chakra, *Sahastara*, the **crown chakra**, information center for our being. Its color is luminescent purple or clear white. It includes the pineal gland. The pineal gland responds to light and darkness and guides our rhythms.

Breathe into the luminescent pearly light of the crown chakra. It contains the unity of humanity and divinity, the integration of human life into cosmic life. Here you will find your own personal experience of the universe, your own connection to your spiritual self, your own way of connecting heaven and earth.

Breathe in and out of your crown chakra. Visualize the vibrations entering and leaving your open skull. Contemplate your true human nature and recognize yourself on this earth. Let loose any vibrations that no longer aid you. Allow the tasks and responsibilities of life to be your best opportunities for growth.

Whether you have visited a few or many chakras, complete your journey by breathing through your entire spine and by visualizing or imagining all your chakras.

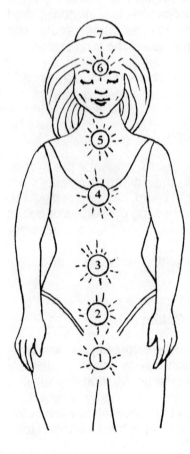

Briefly sense the different vibrations of each chakra. Let your breath stream into and out of every energy center; let your breath move everywhere. With every exhalation imagine that you're giving away everything that you don't need any more. Allow yourself to become free for the new. With every inhalation imagine yourself filling up with the love and healing energies of the universe.

See yourself as whole/ healthy/holy.

Accept yourself your being, your nature, and enjoy yourself as you truly are. Let your joy radiate into the world.

When you are ready, stretch yourself into a sprawl, open your eyes, return to ordinary time and space, and awaken back into your very own life, and your divine humanness.

Fire

Fire cannot be overlooked; it is recognizable from afar. Fire radiates and displays itself; it shows itself boldly. Fire is warmth and fire is light. Fire purifies and burns down: from the ashes arises the Phoenix. I connect fire with the direction of the south, with the summer, tropical fruits, maturity, and abundance. To me, fire is energy, eruption, eros, and willfulness. Aries, Leo and Sagittarius are the astrological fire signs.

To get in touch with fire, I use colors, bold images, and collages.

Color

Colors are healing energies. Colors influence our moods and our vibratory well-being with their different frequencies. Some colors seem cool, others, warm; some seem clear, others hazy. When we utilize the healing properties of colors and bring them into our daily lives, we make their energies our own.

Here are some headstrong, exciting, fun ways to add color to your healing journey.

Play with Colors

Find your own colors. Discover the colors of your own inner fire. Do not seize anything; allow the fire to transform, to burn down the old so that the new can emerge. Meditate about your spectrum of colors. Each color has many properties. Recognize the personal messages for yourself in each color. Forget what you have learned, or read in books or been told about color. You possess enough sense of color yourself. Live it! When you browse through different books on the meanings of color, you will see that different authors assign different colors to the chakras or to the days of the week. You have the same right to invent your own. Play with colors; enjoy them. Look out into nature and discover her colors. Visit a museum and be inspired by the colorful images and objects (and even by the other visitors). "Walk in beauty," say the Navajo. Let color be part of your beauty.

Colors of the Days of the Week

In many languages the names of the days are versions of the name of a goddess or a god or a planet, which, in turn, are associated with specific colors.

Sunday is the day of the sun. Its colors are radiant gold, yellow, orange or white. Sun colors are rich and intense. Use Sun colors to promote serenity and ease, and to open your heart.

Monday is the day of the moon. Its colors are silver or cool blue, occasionally pink. Moon colors are gentle and tender. Use Moon colors to help you become soft and to help guide you through your emotions.

Tuesday, French *mardi*, Spanish *martes,* is the day of Mars, god of war, planet of fierce power. In Swiss German this day is called Zyschtig. According to legend is named after Ziu, another martial god. Its colors are all shades of red. Mars colors are fierce and aggressive. Use Mars colors when you are ready for action. Beware of quarrels, aggressiveness, and pugnacity. Red cannot be ignored.

Weed note: In matrifocal cultures, red is associated with creative, vital energy, not aggression. Red is the color of menstrual blood and birthing blood, not the color of battlefield blood, sacrifice blood. I use the color red when I want to lift my spirits and increase my energy.

Wednesday, French *mercredi*, Spanish *miercoles,* is the day of Mercury, the divine messenger, or Wotan, in Norse traditions. Its colors are turquoise, light yellow, linden green or orange. All sparkly, bright colors belong to Mercury. Use Mercury colors when you travel, when you want to get your message across, and when you hope for change.

Thursday, French *jeudi*, Spanish *jueves*, is the day of Thor or Jupiter, a benevolent, open-hearted, jovial fellow. Its colors are blue-violet, and green. Jupiter colors are very strong and bright. Use Jupiter colors when you want to strengthen your ability to see on the brighter side of life.

Friday, French *vendredi*, Spanish *viernes*, is the day of Freya or Venus. Her colors are rose, pink, sky blue, and apricot. Pastel hues are under the protection of Venus. Use Venus colors to support your female qualities and to heal your sexual energies.

Saturday, is the day of Saturn, planet of hard work and difficult tasks, strength and melancholy. What colors are more befitting than dark green, black, and brown? Saturn colors are deep and rich. But clear white belongs here as well. Saturn helps us distinguish between yes and no, day and night. Use Saturn colors when you wish to pass a threshold or initiate a change in yourself.

Collages

Collages are images which are glued together (from the French *coller*, to glue). Images impress us, reveal us, connect us to our wordless deep selves. Making a collage gives us a time to play with images and to choose images which attract us and speak for us. When we make collages, we create our own compositions in shapes and colors. Collage making helps us see how strongly we are affected by the images we consume. Images reverberate for a long time in our souls. Do you pay attention to the images that you absorb? Do you consume random images? what TV delivers? From the images we receive each day, we create our dreams, like a living collage. Is it not of great significance, then, what we choose to take into ourselves and preserve in our innermost spaces?

Women at my workshops create collages and over and over I see them discover with astonishment clues to particular mysterious moods revealed in those (often hastily thrown together) collages. Suddenly they recognize the hole into which they were just about to fall. Or they see, with surprise, what is hindering them in the expression of their true individuality. Dreams reveal themselves in these collages as well, sometimes with much more clarity than words allow.

When we show our collages to each other and discuss our images, amazing new insights are often revealed. Listening to the opinions of others reflecting on our choice of images helps us discover many new things about ourselves.

To begin your collage, collect old magazines, paste and a big sheet of blank paper. Choose a theme, such as: "What does being a woman mean to me?" and look for fitting images: symbols, headlines, advertising. Tear or cut out these treasures.

Lay them on your large paper, sliding them around until you've created a new image from the individual pieces that feels just right to you. It is best not to think much; let the unconscious emerge unaltered. Glue makes your collage permanent.

When you are done, share your collage with friends, or use your collage as the focus of your meditation. If you create different collages over the course of time and then look at them chronologically, you will delight yourself with insights.

Weed note: The value of art therapy—whether it be through collages, clay, or paint—is in its ability to tap into the pre-verbal levels of our experiences. Many of our detrimental attitudes about ourselves, especially in relation to our sex-roles, are absorbed before we can speak. Art therapy allows us to change these attitudes at deep levels of the psyche.

We also absorb the disconnected, disempowered images of women relentlessly thrust at us by the magazines, television, movies, and videos of the dominant culture.When we consciously choose to change the way we think and feel about ourselves, these images—like hidden snares—can trap us and frustrate us. Art therapy releases these snares and allows to change as we envision.

Earth

On Earth we live. She carries us. She attracts us. We all obey her gravity. Earth is deep. She connects us all. For me the Earth is matter, the north. She is firm, yet fertile. Taurus, Virgo, and Capricorn are the astrological signs of the Earth element.

We come from the Earth and return to her. "The Earth is our Mother," say the Native American people, while the Holy Bible proclaims the opposite: "Thou shalt make Earth your subject." How can we come to a wise exchange with our Earth? How can we take what we need and not abuse the environment? I've seen Native Americans and wise women who ask permission or give a gift before they take something from Earth, for instance, a plant. To me, this is one way to honor Earth, to show equality with everything surrounding us, to acknowledge that many beings share this Earth and this life with us.

When I want to connect with the energies of Earth, I reach for whatever is palpable or tangible: fresh food, textured fabrics, fat candles. Scent, too, such as smudge from cedar or sage, helps me open to Earth energies.

Here are a few earthy suggestions from my own experiences to get you started in this realm. And, of course, as always, I encourage you to invent and go on your own journeys of discovery as you contact and experience Earth.

Food

"Food keeps body and soul together," says a German proverb. How true.

"You are what you eat." I consist of what I take in, transform, and make into myself. The process of taking nourishment and giving nourishment is a constant process of life on earth, and when we do it, we change, we transform. Utter alchemy!

When we really become aware of this, we choose real (not processed) foods and arrive naturally at healthy eating habits far away from dogmas, diets, or the dictates of fashion. We can allow ourselves, like animals, to use our instinct for what we need and for how much we need.

Weed note: Only true if we do not surround ourselves with soda and chips and oversweetened fake foods. Even if you think you have lost this instinct, you can revive it again.

A good method to stir up your instinct and help you recognize your needs is a very short break from eating. I take a day free of food now and then to sharpen my senses for what my metabolism needs. Instead of eating, I listen to my desires. This is said easily and yet it is often so hard to do. It is difficult to trust my inner wisdom for I am used to trusting science more than myself. To dig up my intuition again, to unearth it and to renew my faith in it, is an exciting undertaking. I cannot teach you how to do this, only encourage you to do it. No book, no advice, no workshop will help. The ability to trust in your inner voice can only be learned by you, by, well, just trusting it! Have courage!

Here are a few things my intuition has told me. Maybe they will help you, or jiggle your intuition when you need help with these following reproductive organ problems.

Foods That Prevent Menstrual Cramps

To help prevent pain before and during the menses, try eating less animal products. Animal proteins and animal fats are hard to digest and can contribute to erratic, abnormal hormone production. I stick to a vegetarian diet, or even a diet of raw vegetables if the menstrual cramps are intense.

Weed note: The most critical nutrient for preventing cramps in any muscle, including the uterus, is calcium. Eat at least a cup of organic milk, yogurt or low-fat cheese every day for a week before you bleed and watch those cramps disappear. Nonorganic dairy and meat is loaded with hormones and best avoided. Peppermint, comfrey leaves, stinging nettle, seaweed and oatstraw are superb calcium sources.

Fertility Foods

My favorite fertility-increasing foods (recommended for both women and men) are sesame seeds, honey, almonds, rose blossoms and leaves, passion fruit and passion flower, peonies, and sour milk products such as yogurt, buttermilk, kefir, whey, curds, quark, cottage cheese, ricotta and the like.

Watch out for the fertility-decreasing effects of coffee and bean sprouts. If you need a cuppa something to help you wake up in the morning, try grain coffee. Sprouts from any beans, including alfalfa sprouts, mung beans sprouts, and lentil sprouts, inhibit fertility. This was first observed in animals grazing on such plants.

Weed note: Carrots also inhibit fertility, especially when juiced. For healthy babies, mom and dad need to eat plenty of foods rich in folic acid, like all leafy greens, and foods rich in vitamin E, like sunflower seeds, before conception. Though it is a member of the bean family, red clover is the best fertility enhancer I've ever come across.

Foods That Prevent PMS

To help prevent premenstrual problems, I eat foods very rich in vitamins E and C. For vitamin E, I eat whole grains, seeds, sprouts, and shoots, and wheat germ oil. For vitamin C, I eat fresh fruits, especially citrus, parsley, and fresh green salad. Some Australian women I know find that eating lots of onions and garlic eliminates PMS discomfort. I consider it better to eat foods with these vitamins than to take vitamin supplements.

Fabric

Have you experienced the healing effects of fabric? Cloths of various textures, woven, knit or tied together, can be very sensual, very earthy, very comforting. What kinds of materials colors and shapes do you wear? Each fabric has a life and a story. Some will agree with you more than others.

The lanolin in raw wool, triggers allergic reactions in some people. Cotton, linen, ramie, and rayon are plant fibers that rarely cause allergic reactions. Unfortunately they are often treated chemically to make them more durable, or softer, or wrinkle-free, or fire-resistant. Formaldehyde is a common dressing agent for these "natural fiber" fabrics. That's why I thoroughly wash new clothes before the first wearing.

Are you comfortable with furs and leather? The vibration of animal skins has a special healing energy, but some people dislike the thought of using something from a dead animal.

Do you wear silk? In commercial silk production, a living being is killed: the silkworm. That worm dreams of becoming a butterfly as it pupates in its cocoon. Instead, it is thrown into boiling water, and dies. This produces long, durable silk threads, rather than the short, rough threads formed when the silkworm butterfly chews its way out of the cocoon.

Weed note: Silk is the fabric of protection. Silk stops vibrations. I wear silk when I have to spend time in hospitals, TV stations, or crowds.

Fabric Acupuncture

If you don't like acupuncture needles, try fabric acupuncture. Cut small pieces of silk and place them on acupoints. Different colors and shapes create different effects. Cool colors are calming, warm colors are stimulating. Circular patches are relaxing, square ones increase active participation in the world. Triangles have a balancing effect.

Weed note: Use a paste made from plain white flour and a little water to "glue" your fabric patches onto your skin if you wish to be active while the healing treatment goes on. Or lie down and have someone else place the fabric acupuncture on you, weighing the fabric patches down with various crystals and semi-precious stones to magnify and potentize the healing energies.

Scents

We take in scents with our nose. The nose and the sense of smell is associated with the Earth element in Yoga. I enjoy creating and influencing my moods with scents. To add scent to my life, I use incense sticks, aromatherapy lamps, and naturally scented massage oils.

Incense sticks add the fire element to the Earth energy. Aromatherapy lamps bring all elements into space and time: a bowl of pottery or metal (*Earth*) is filled with *water* and a few drops of essential oil are added. A candle (*fire* and *earth*) underneath heats the oil and disperses the scent as the water evaporates into the *air*.

When we anoint ourselves with lovely smells, we take in the aroma through our pores as well as our nose. A scented body oil massaged into the skin seizes us completely. I urge you to use natural essential oils rather than cheaper synthetic perfume extracts as the healing (or harmful) qualities of scent are profound and some people react very badly to synthetic smells.

Here are my favorite ways to help myself with scent:

Aromatherapy For Pain

When I have menstrual cramps or want to feel calm, I choose the essential oil of rose. I find it very relaxing. Rosemary essential oil is analgesic (pain-relieving) and energizing. The smell of fresh ginger or ginger oil is said to relieve pain and have a harmonizing effect, balancing and evening out energies.

Weed note: Ginger compresses are a classic remedy from the Orient for treating sore muscles and any pain from congested tissues. Essential oil of cedar is a safe, mild soother for pain.

Aromatherapy to Stimulate Fertility

The essential oils which stimulate fertility are Musk, Ginger, Vanilla, Patchouli, Ylang-Ylang, Cinnamon, Cloves, Geranium, and Basil. You can also try using more basil, cloves, ginger, cinnamon, and vanilla in your cooking to heighten sexual pleasure and increase your chances of conceiving.

Aromatherapy For Relaxation or Stimulation

When I want help to retreat from my daily stresses I choose Jasmine, Birch, Lavender, Rose, Cypress, or Cedar Wood for my scent. When I need to have lots of energy, I choose one of these scents: Rosemary, Geranium, Bergamot, Basil, or Juniper.

Weed note: DO NOT USE ESSENTIAL OILS ON THE SKIN unless you dilute them and test your skin to see if it is reactive. DO NOT TAKE ESSENTIAL OILS INTERNALLY. Store essential oils under lock and key if there are young children in your house. Consuming even 1/2 ounce of essential oil can be fatal.

Candles

Candles stimulate our fire by their burning, but through their material they also connect us to the earth. Wax can come from petroleum or be created by bees in their hives. It brings the malleable, yet firm qualities of the earth close to us. Candles can be anointed with essential oils so they give off scents as they burn, aiding our journey into the earth of our being. (See previous aromatherapy suggestions.) Candles can take us to our dreams and candles can ground us as well. (See page 167 for ideas about candle colors.)

Weed note: I use candles every day to help me. Candles provide light that is superbly relaxing to my nervous system. Candles bring the elements of earth, fire, and air right into my living space. Candles help me send blessings, healing energies, and prayers. Candles remind me to focus my intent and give me an easy way to do it.

When I want fast action on my intention, I burn several small candles. When I want endurance and steadfast action for my intention, I choose a large candle and let it remain burning for many hours (or even days). When I want to sweeten my intention, I light a beeswax candle.

When I want to attract abundance, I use gold candles or green candles. When I want passion, nothing but red candles, preferably the kind that drip, will do. I honor the fertility of the dark moon with black candles; time to begin, to spin anew. I honor the letting go of the full moon with white candles; time to surrender.

The Most Important Element :
Human Interaction

In addition to the four elements and four directions, there is the Center, from which everything originates. The elements of earth, air, fire, and water are not in a void without reference; they are related to us, they affect us as human beings. The center is the place of interaction.

I want to tell you how especially important human interaction has been to me in my healing journey. What distinguishes us from animals is not only our work or our tears of joy and pain, but the special interactions human beings have through different kinds of language, and our ability to understand each other and express compassion.

When we exchange and share ourselves with one another, there is healing. When we communicate, entering into dialogue with others or with ourselves, there is healing. Conversations, sitting together, even upsetting one another, brings us closer toward ourselves and to one another.

In every human interaction, we can discover something about other people and learn something about ourselves, whether we are arguing against one another or just casually meeting someone. We strengthen our connections with all of life when we discover that others feel similarly. We expand our consciousness and our view of the world when we learn that others feel differently. When I share my experiences with LUNA YOGA I not only teach others but also find new aspects to consider in my own ongoing practice.

I consider self-communication as important as communication with others. To understand different parts in myself aids me in understanding others. Finding ways to be gentle and loving with myself helps me be more compassionate toward others.

Letting go of my grandiose principles and dictating dogmas frees me from the rigidity of my own system and frees up my relationships to others. I use the I Ching, the Tarot, and my journal to help me understanding myself.

When logical thinking is no further help, I reach for the Tarot; its images contribute new, nonverbal, ways of looking at myself and my life. When I feel stuck, I ask the I Ching, the ancient Chinese Book of Changes, a question, knowing that it will tell me that nothing is permanent, even what is considered good or bad is constantly changing. When I feel out of the rhythms of my life, out of the rhythms of nature, these tools help me talk to myself.

My journal serves as a guide into the depths of myself. In my journal I capture what moves me, I describe my different moods, I discover my own inner cycles. When I sit and reflect on my day, remembering what was significant and writing it down, I receive clues to myself, or sometimes a lightning flash of insight. I learn about my own inner truths, how they change like the moon, yet lose nothing of their stability.

This poem from the Upanishads describes it beautifully:

We know that milk
has always the same color,
although the cows that give it,
are colored differently.
Likewise the wisdom is one,
although the doctrines might differ,
just as the color of milk is one,
although the cows differ.
And wisdom is in the depth of each individual hidden
like within milk is the butter that we don't see.
Therefore the wise practitioner has to accomplish
the churning within that is necessary for making butter,
while consciousness should without hesitation
take on the role of ferment.

Amrtabindu Upanishad I 18-20

LUNA YOGA

PART SIX

ENDINGS & BEGINNINGS

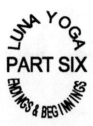

LUNA YOGA
PART SIX
ENDINGS & BEGINNINGS

Utopia: A Visionary Dream

In the evening I read a poem by the East Indian philosopher Rabindranath Tagore. In the morning I awoke with the following lines:

On the shore of endless times
people meet:
wander along peacefully,
dance, leap, laugh,
cry and grieve.
They run and jump,
pause and gaze;
everything is possible.
They listen to the waves, to the storm.
It is summer and winter.
Mountains in snow.
Rivers meander over the land.

On the shore of endless worlds
heaven and earth meet.
A volcano spews fire.
Spring awakens.
Autumn sends leaves.
The earth trembles.
The weather revives.

On the shore of endless cycles
life and death meet:
Phoenix rises from the ashes.
Red morning sky changes into sunset.
Dying passes, life arises,
creation takes place.

On the shore of endless earths
people meet:
children, women, men,
animals among them,
plants of all kinds in
different stages of growth.

Is it the paradise of far-away imagination?
No. It is Utopia,
in which more is possible than peace and solemn silence:
everything finds its place,
transforms itself,
changes like the moon.

On the shore of endless dreams
all meet
and play their game,
consciously alive
with clarity, serenity and power.
They have discovered their moods,
experience them lively, embodied
as the offering of natural gifts.

On the shore of endless utopias
we meet
and exchange ourselves,
enjoy the encounter
and walk in beauty
to our task.

Thanking and Rejoicing

I am filled with joy today: joy about completing this book, joy about my freedom, joy about work finished well. I am filled with joy about my own creativity and about all that has been nourished and will be nourished by my words and my work.

I offer thanks to:
My women friends, old and new,
My men friends here and there,
My former housemates in Munich and
My current house community in Biel.

I offer thanks to:
My teachers, for guiding me along the steps of my path.
The many different people in my workshops who inspired me.
The Sky and Earth, who were favorable toward me,
as well as the Stars, the Sun, and most certainly, the Moon.

I offer special thanks to:
Raimund Thomas of Munich, who financed the LUNA YOGA drawings by Esther Lisette Ganz.

My farewell is this text from an old book on TantraYoga:

*This body serves for pleasures of the world
and for liberation of the Yogi,
who resembles the grove of a sage.
Your own body is like a metropolis,
serving the experience of highest bliss,
not of suffering.
Like an experienced charioteer skillfully directs the chariot,
this body, too, must not be treated thoughtlessly.
Like a fired clay doll can be broken by a child,
thus this wholesome body can be destroyed by
consciousness in a wink,
when it commits harmful acts of will.*

Yoga-Vasistha IV.23.2.X 44-45

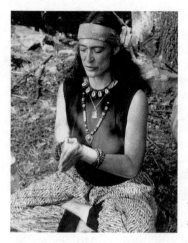

Susun Weed is the editor-in-chief of Ash Tree Publishing. She began practicing yoga 30 years ago, just about the time she started studying herbal medicine. Her purpose in starting a publishing house was two-fold: to provide women with empowering information about health care, and to connect women's health with women's spirituality. Susun is the voice of the Wise Woman Tradition and a friend of the fairies.

*I especially wish to thank my friend **Betsy Sandlin**. First, for introducing me to the study of Yoga; second, for her personal example of the fertility-modulating effects of Yoga; and, most importantly, for her dedication to excellence in the proofreading and editing of the American version of LUNA YOGA.*

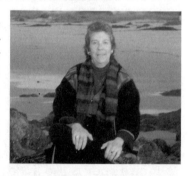

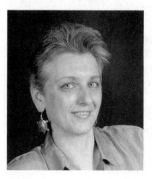

Meret Liebenstein has been dedicated to the study of natural healing and women's health for all of her adult life. She studied LUNA YOGA with Adelheid Ohlig in Germany before coming to America in 1988. *Translating LUNA YOGA fulfilled my dream of utilizing my language skills and bicultural experience to contribute to the world-wide movement to reclaim Wise Woman ways.*

Adelheid Ohlig is the creator of LUNA YOGA. She works as a freelance journalist in Europe, especially in her home country Switzerland, in addition to spending much of her time teaching LUNA YOGA to women who wish to control their own reproductive health with minimal use of chemicals, hormones and surgery. Adelheid's story, and her obvious skill as a yoga teacher impressed Susun as soon as they met, and Susun promptly arranged to bring LUNA YOGA, and Adelheid's wisdom, to American women.

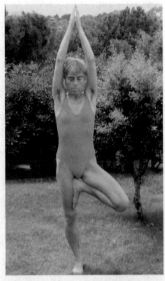

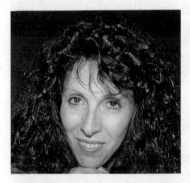

Amy Sophia Marashinsky, is Girl Friday at Ash Tree Publishing. She is better known as an award-winning filmmaker, writer/director/producer of theatre, author, and drummer. She conducts Shamanic-Priestess Apprenticeships from her home in the Northeast.

Kimberley Eve currently lives in rural N.Y. She works as in-house-artist for Ash Tree Publishing. Her flip-side career is as an entertainer for children at parties and fairs. Since working on LUNA YOGA, Kimberley has added several new postures to her regular practice.

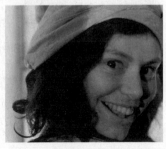

Resources and Further Reading

Fertility

Conscious Conception, Parvati-Baker, Baker & Slayton, Freestone, 1986

The Fertility Awareness Handbook, Barbara Kass-Annese, Hunter House

Lunar Calendar, $1.50, Snake & Snake, Rt 3 Box 165, Durham, NC 27713

Healthy/Healing/Wholing

Acupressure Way Of Health: Jin Shin Do, Teeguarden, Japan Pub, 1978

The Body Has Its Reasons: Self-Awareness with Conscious Movement, Therese Bertherat and Carol Bemstein, Healing Arts, 1989

Cooperative Method of Natural Birth Control, Margaret Nofziger, Book Publishing Company, 1991

Energy Ecstacy: Your Seven Vital Chakras), B. Gunther, Newcastle, 1983

Faces of the Moon Mother, Rowena Pattee Kryder, Golden Point, 1991

Gyn/Ecology, Mary Daly, Beacon Press, 1978

Hands of Light, Barbara Brennan, Bantam, 1987

Healing Wise: Second Wise Woman Herbal, Susun Weed, Ash Tree, 1989

Hygieia: A Woman's Herbal, Jeannine Parvati, Freestone Collective, 1978

Inner Bridges: A Guide to Energy Movement and Body Structure, Fritz Frederick Smith, M.D., Humanics New Age, 1986

Joy of Feeling: Bodymind Acupressure, Iona Marsaa Teeguarden, Japan Pub, 1984

Life Tuning with Primal Sounds: Chakra Music, A. Keyserling & R. Losey, School of Wisdom, 1993

Listening to our Bodies: The Rebirth of Feminine Wisdom, Stephanie Demetralopoulos, Beacon Press, 1983

Mother Wit: A Guide to Healing and Psychic Development, Diane Mariechild, Crossing Press, 1988

Motherpeace: A Way to the Goddess through Myth, Art and Tarot, Vickie Noble, Harper, 1983

Mysteries of the Dark Moon, Demetra George, Harper, 1992

New View of A Woman's Body, Carol Downer, ed., Federation of Feminist Health Centers, Simon & Shuster, 1991

Natural Healing In Gynecology, Rina Nissim, Pandora, 1986

Opening the Heart of the Womb (audio), Ondrea and Stephen Levine, 4 Cielo Ln., #4, Novato, CA 94949

Qi Gong: Ancient Chinese Way to Health, Dong & Esser, Paragon, 1990

Reflexology for Women, Nicola Hall, Harper, 1994

Second Book Of DO-IN: Rejuvenation through Self-Massage, Jacques de Langre, Happiness Press, 1974

Wheels of Life, Anodea Judith, Llewellyn, 1987

Working on Yourself Alone, Arnold Mindell, Arkana, 1990

Sex

Art of Sexual Ecstasy, Margo Anand, Tarcher, 1991

Cultivating Female Sexual Energy, Manweewan Chia, Healing Tao, 1986

Deep Down: New Sensual Writing by Women, Laura Chester, ed., Faber and Faber, 1989

*E*ve's Garden, Catalog $3, 119 W. 57th St., Suite 14206, NY, NY 10019

Female Ejaculation, How to do it! (video), Fanny Fatale, $34.95, Fatale Videos, 526 Castro St., San Francisco, CA 94114

Ladies Own Erotica, Kensington Ladies' Erotica Society, Ten Speed Press, 1984

The Love Muscle: Every Woman's Guide to Intensifying Sexual Pleasure, Bryce Britton, Signet /NAL, 1982

Riding Desire: An Anthology of Erotic Writing, Tee Corinne, ed., Banned Books, 1991

Sex for One: The Joy of Self-Loving, Betty Dodson, Crown, 1992

Sex Over Forty Newsletter, POBox 1600, Chapel Hill, NC 27515

Sexuality Library for Women, catalog $2, Open Enterprises, 1210 Valencia, San Francisco, CA 94110

Self-loving (video), Betty Dodson, $45, Box 1933, Murray Hill Station, NY, NY 10156

Slow Hand: Women Writing Erotica, Michele Slung, ed., Harper, 1993

Tantra (magazine), POBox 79, Torreon, NM 87061, $4.50 sample

Women's Mysteries

Dragon Time: Magic And Mystery Of Menstruation, Luisa Francia, Ash Tree, 1991

Blessings of the Blood, Celu Amberston, Beach Holme, 1991

Blood Magic, Buckley & Gottlieb, University of California Press, 1983

Her Blood is Gold: Celebrating The Power of Menstruation, Lara Owen, Harper, 1993

Herbal Healing for Women, Rosemary Gladstar, Fireside, 1993

Menopausal Years The Wise Woman Way, Susun Weed, Ash Tree, 1992

Moon, Moon, Anne Kent Rush, Random House, 1976 (out of print)

Moon Time (audio) and *Moon Lodge* (audio), Brooke Medicine Eagle, Harmony Network, POBox 2550, Guerneville, CA 95446

Red Flower: Rethinking Menstruation, Dena Taylor, Crossing Press, 1988

Self-Ritual for Invoking Release of Spirit Life in the Womb, ($6), Deborah Maia, Mother Spirit Publishing, POBox 893, Great Barrington, MA 01230

Shakti Woman, Vicki Noble, Harper, 1991

Songs of Bleeding, Spider, Black Thistle Press, 1992

Sister Moon Lodge: The Power and Mystery of Menstruation, Kisma K. Stepanish, Llewellyn, 1992

Wise Wound: Myths, Realities And Meanings Of Menstruation, Penelope Shuttle and Peter Redgrove, Grove Press, 1986

Wise Woman Herbal for Childbearing Year, Susun Weed, Ash Tree, 1985

Yoga

Awakening the Spine, Vanda Scaravelli, Harper, 1991

Ecstasy through Tantra, Jonn Mumford, Llewellyn Pub., 1987

Learn Yoga In A Weekend, Sivananda Yoga Vedanta Center Staff, Knopf, 1993

Sivananda Companion To Yoga, Sivananda Yoga Center, Simon & Schuster, 1983

Some Still Want the Moon, Vimala McClure, Nucleus Publications, 1989

Yoga, a Gem for Women, Geeta Iyengar, Timeless, 1983

Yoga For A Better Life: How To Compose Your Own Complete Yoga Course, David Schonfeld, Quest, 1980

Yoga for a New Age, Bob Smith and Linda Boudreau Smith, Smith Productions, 1986

Yoga, the Iyengar Way, Silva, Mira & Shyam Mehta, Knopf, 1994

Yoga Journal, 2054 University Ave., Berkeley, CA 94704

Yoga International Magazine, Rural Route 1, Box 407, Honesdale, PA 18431

Essential Oils

Aromatherapy for Women, Maggie Tisserand, Healing Arts, 1985

Essential Oil Co., PO Box 88, Sandy, OR 97055; (503) 695-2400

Aromalamp, 369 Montezuma, #111, Sante Fe, NM 87501 (800-933-5267)